Vegetarian Ketogenic
COOKBOOK FOR BEGINNERS

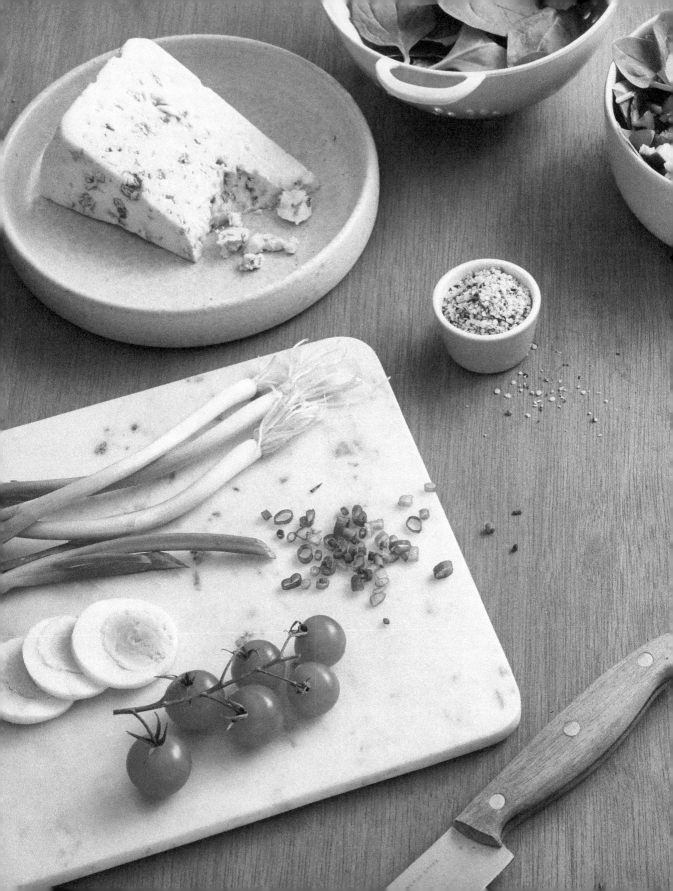

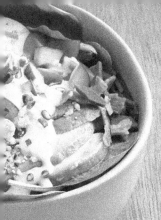

Vegetarian
Ketogenic

COOKBOOK FOR BEGINNERS

75 Recipes and a 14-Day Meal Plan for Healthy Living

Alicia Shevetone

R

ROCKRIDGE
PRESS

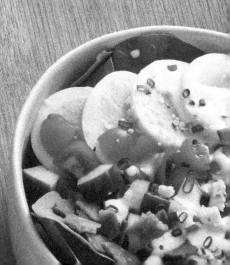

For general information on our other products and services or to obtain technical support, please contact our Customer Care Department within the United States at (866) 744-2665, or outside the United States at (510) 253-0500.

Rockridge Press publishes its books in a variety of electronic and print formats. Some content that appears in print may not be available in electronic books, and vice versa.

TRADEMARKS: Rockridge Press and the Rockridge Press logo are trademarks or registered trademarks of Callisto Media Inc. and/or its affiliates, in the United States and other countries, and may not be used without written permission. All other trademarks are the property of their respective owners. Rockridge Press is not associated with any product or vendor mentioned in this book.

Interior and Cover Designer: Patricia Fabricant
Art Producer: Hannah Dickerson
Editor: Marjorie DeWitt
Production Editor: Ruth Sakata Corley
Production Manager: Michael Kay

Photography © 2021 Annie Martin, cover; © Biz Jones, back cover (top) and p. 20; © Darren Muir, back cover (center) and pp. X, 50, 64, 94, 106, 120; © Nadine Greeff, back cover (bottom) and p. 82; © Laura Flippen, pp. II-III, 36; © Evi Abeler, p. VI

Paperback ISBN: 978-1-63807-308-6 |
eBook ISBN: 978-1-63807-213-3
R0

*To my cherished husband, Mark,
and the macro/micro balance
we've shared for 25 years.*

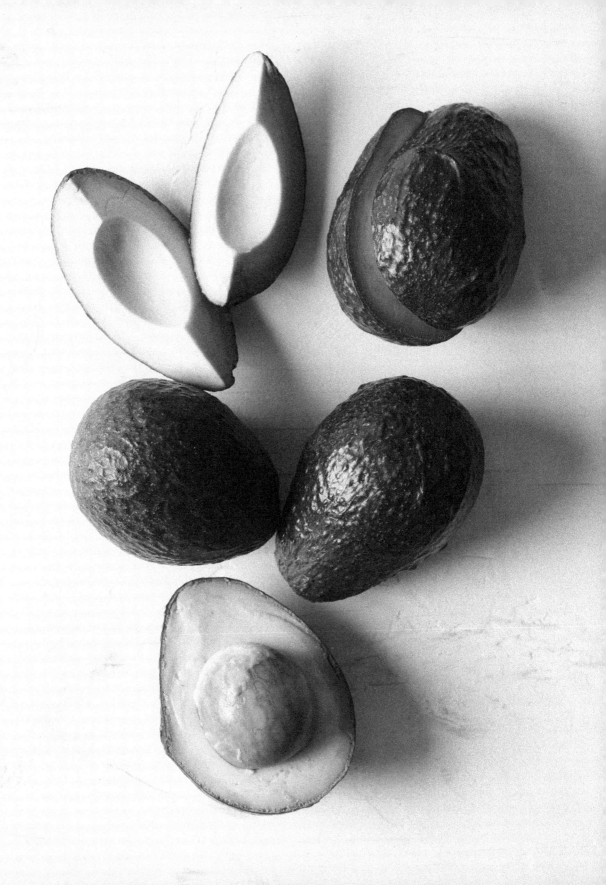

Contents

INTRODUCTION viii

CHAPTER 1   Keto, the Vegetarian Way 1
            14-DAY MEAL PLAN.. 14

CHAPTER 2   Breakfast and Beverages.................................. 21

CHAPTER 3   Salads and Sandwiches 37

CHAPTER 4   Soups, Stews, and Chilis.................................. 51

CHAPTER 5   Mains.. 65

CHAPTER 6   Snacks.. 83

CHAPTER 7   Desserts 95

CHAPTER 8   Homemade Staples..107

            MEASUREMENT CONVERSIONS 121
            INDEX 122

Introduction

We might not know each other very well just yet—but, hello! I'm Alicia. I think we'll get along because I, too, am intrigued by ketogenic and vegetarian cuisines. Actually, the three of us go way back. Before I even knew the dietary significance of carbohydrates (circa 2007), one of my friends told me that she was able to stay slim if she had "less than 40 net carbs per day." Ever the optimist, I thought, "How hard could it be?" From that point forward, I realized that any lifestyle that not only supported, but actually encouraged, my lifelong obsession with dairy had to have significant merit. And so my ketogenic fascination began.

A couple years later, a dietary malaise set in—the culinary equivalent of a melancholy I couldn't quite articulate. I started reading books like Alicia Silverstone's *The Kind Diet*, Kathy Freston's *Veganist*, and Mark Bittman's *How to Cook Everything Vegetarian*. Although I had no desire to completely convert to vegetarianism, the realization that eating meat-free meals just a few times per week could have a profound and positive impact on my health, as well as the sustainability of our planet, offered me a renewed optimism and comfort that I couldn't ignore. Ever since, I've described myself as someone with "vegetarian tendencies."

Despite my heart being in the right place, it was often challenging to reconcile traditionally meat-forward keto meals with my burgeoning interest in vegetarian dishes, especially at the beginning. At first, I wasn't sure they were even scientifically compatible, let alone tasty companions. After minimal investigation and some R&D in my kitchen, I began to discover that keto and vegetarian cuisines aren't mutually exclusive. They not only play well together but are a brilliant match that takes no more effort to cook than any other combination of ingredients. All the details you need to start this journey are contained in the pages of this book.

The book is structured with ease in mind. The first order of business is to offer you an introduction to the vegetarian keto lifestyle, including the ingredients and basic kitchen tools you'll need. I'll then answer some frequently asked questions and give you some tips for making this way of life simple and practical to follow. Next, you'll find a 14-day meal plan—two weeks of breakfasts, lunches, and dinners, featuring a variety of Quick, One-Pot, and 5-Ingredient recipes to jump-start your new regimen. The remaining chapters provide 75 beginner-friendly vegetarian keto recipes, organized from Breakfast through Dessert, including Homemade Staples you'll use throughout.

Soon, you will develop the confidence to swap out non-keto-friendly ingredients, insert vegetables where there were none before, and even create new vegetarian keto recipes using your favorite produce and pantry items. And if you get stuck, look me up on social media. There's nothing I enjoy more than supporting kindred spirits on their quest for scrumptious food (except, maybe, eating it). Until then, enjoy this new adventure and all the savory tastes it has to offer—cheers!

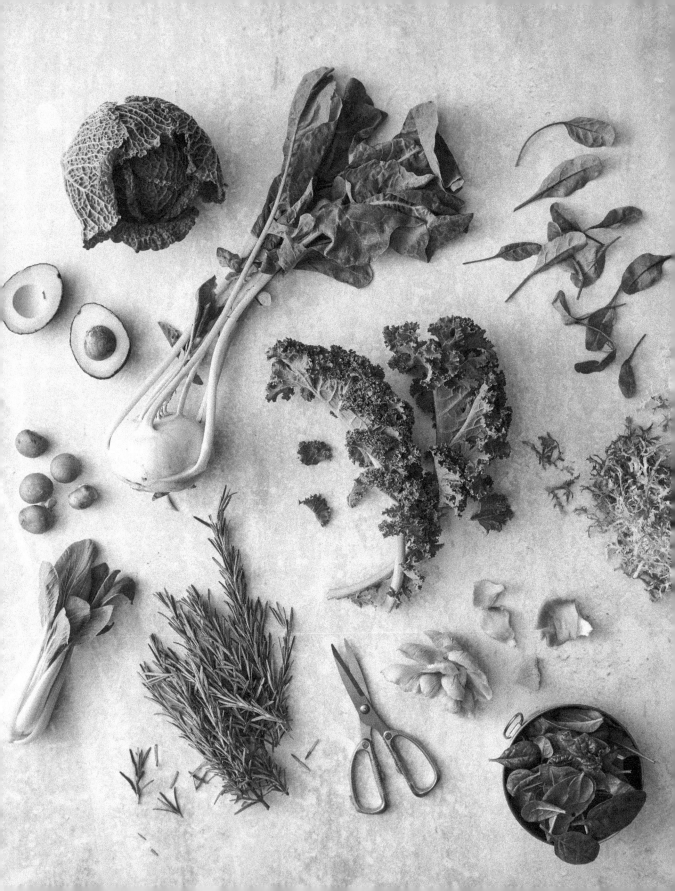

CHAPTER 1

Keto, the Vegetarian Way

Your keto vegetarian journey is about to begin. In this chapter, I'll explain the basics of ketosis, including macronutrients and micronutrients, and the foods that will help you stay on track. We'll cover some easy steps to help define your goals and set you up for success in reaching them. You will also learn some simple tips to help you find your keto-vegetarian groove, including your very own 14-day meal plan.

Keto Without Meat?

Whether you currently follow a vegetarian diet, a ketogenic lifestyle, both, or neither, this book will guide you along your journey toward improved health, weight loss, and sustainable maintenance. You might be familiar with the traditional keto diet, which allows for protein (including meat and seafood) and high-fat and low-carbohydrate foods. This book follows the keto diet as it intersects with the standard lacto-ovo vegetarian diet, which primarily consists of grains, vegetables, fruit and nuts, some eggs and dairy, and no animal protein.

Plant-based and keto diets are both widespread in popularity. Although each is very effective as a singular strategy, the fusion of the two dramatically accelerates your dietary impact, including a number of health benefits.

Increased fat burning. By reducing sugar and carbohydrate intake, your body pivots from burning glucose to burning fat. This process is referred to as ketosis, which enables weight loss.

Weight loss. We all want to look our best; however, safe weight loss using a vegetarian ketogenic diet also greatly reduces strain on your joints and vital organs, reduces cancer risk, and lowers cholesterol.

More energy. Plant protein is easier for the body to break down than animal protein. Less energy to metabolize your food means more energy available to fuel your day.

Improved digestion. Vegetables and fruits are loaded with fiber and good bacteria, and your body will thank you.

Better mood. When your body isn't struggling to digest complex carbohydrates, sleep generally improves. A great night's sleep ensures that you're well rested, clearheaded, and more prepared to navigate day-to-day life.

The typical ketogenic diet is packed with animal protein, which may suggest that keto and vegetarian lifestyles aren't a natural fit. Rest assured, by honoring the primary principles of each diet, you will quickly realize that the intersection of both lifestyles is where you will see the greatest benefits. The tips and recipes in this book will convince you that a vegetarian ketogenic diet is not only logical, it's affordable, sustainable, and tons of fun in the kitchen, too.

Some of the freshest, most delicious vegetarian foods are naturally low in carbohydrates, making them ideal for your ketogenic adventure. All you need to unlock their potential is a plan. Here are five easy steps to follow to ensure your success.

1 **Create your keto goals.** What is your primary motivation? Whether it's losing weight or simply feeling healthier, set your "North Star"—a fixed point that governs your intention and focus. Make it realistic so you can reinforce your optimism on a daily basis and maintain your focus.

2 **Clean out the kitchen.** Later in this chapter, you'll find a list of foods to love, limit, and lose. Use this list as a quick reference guide to determine which ingredients will earn their right to remain on the premises. Collect the foods you need to lose and offer them to friends (or donate them) so they don't go to waste.

3 **Stock up.** As soon as you begin to master what to eat, you'll learn exactly which ingredients you should keep on hand. A well-stocked refrigerator and pantry contain a combination of fresh and shelf-stable items that offer the nutrients you need to achieve your goals. Don't worry, I'll give you a list.

4 **Follow the 14-day meal plan.** Full disclosure: I didn't like meal plans until I created the one in this book. Most meal plans instruct you to cook a limited number of meals in large quantity, which equates to monotony and too many leftovers. My 14-day meal plan is a dynamic guide that takes variety and balance into consideration, because when you love what you're eating, it's easy to stick to the diet.

5 **Establish your routine.** Consistency is critical to embedding the healthy behaviors needed for long-term success. Keep it simple, find meals you love, and make them with someone you love. An accountability partner is invaluable if you have a hard time changing your eating habits.

How Does Keto Work?

If you are new to keto, this section offers you a brief overview to explain the basics. If you've dabbled in keto in the past, some of the following information may be repeat knowledge. In that case, read on for a refresher.

ALL ABOUT MACROS

Keto success is rooted in eating the correct ratio of fat, protein, and carbohydrates. This trifecta is also known as macronutrients, or "macros." Macros deliver the energy, or calories, you need to function optimally. Each macro has a target range to achieve the ideal balance. On the vegetarian keto diet, I advise beginners to shoot for meals that are composed of around 65 percent fat, 20 percent protein, and 15 percent carbohydrates. If you've experimented with a keto diet that includes meat, that carbohydrate number may look high. This is because many vegetables are naturally high in carbohydrates, so vegetarian keto allows for a slightly higher level of carbs than omnivore keto.

Any fiber you consume offsets your carb intake, resulting in what we call "net carbs." For example, one cup of chopped broccoli has 6 grams of total carbs and 2.4 grams of fiber, which works out to 3.6 grams of net carbs.

GETTING INTO KETOSIS

When you digest carbohydrates, your body converts the carbs into glucose. Glucose is essentially sugar, which your body uses for fuel. By migrating to a low-carb diet, you are challenging your body to transition from burning sugar to burning fat and ketones (an alternative fuel your liver produces when it's low on glucose) for energy. This process is called ketosis. Achieving ketosis can take several weeks, even months.

The easiest and most affordable method to confirm whether your body is in ketosis is to use ketone urine strips, which you can find at most pharmacies or online. Their reliability improves with hydration, so be sure to drink plenty of water. It's also recommended that you test your urine at the same time every day.

To stay in ketosis, you'll want to track your macros, keep alcohol consumption to a minimum, and maintain an active lifestyle.

So, how many net carbs, protein, and fat should you consume? Everyone's ideal macros differ, because we all metabolize food at different rates; however, if you're following the 65/20/15 ratio of fat to protein to carbs, that will look something like 160 grams of fat, 65 grams of protein, and 40 grams of net carbs per day.

The key to tracking your macros is knowing how to calculate them. The recipes in this cookbook have been formulated to meet the target ratios, but how will you track your macros out in the real world? If you follow keto bloggers, they almost always list macros for every recipe to confirm it's within range. For me, tracking macros on my phone using an app is the best method. I like MyFitnessPal because it tracks my weight and workouts, as well as what I eat and drink.

There are numerous free online calculators and formulas to calculate just how many calories you should consume, depending on your sex, activity level, height, current weight, and age. Simply enter "formula to track keto macros" into an internet search engine and you will be flooded with options. Once you have that calorie number, the basic formula to calculate your macros is very simple: Take your daily calorie target and multiply by the percentage of each macro as a decimal.

For example, for a 1,500-calorie diet:

- Fat (65%): 0.65 x 1,500 = 975 calories from fat

- Protein (20%): 0.2 x 1,500 = 300 calories from protein

- Carbs (15%): 0.15 x 1,500 = 225 calories from carbohydrates

Weight loss requires a caloric deficit, which means you're burning more calories than you are taking in. For most people, a caloric deficit of 500 calories per day will trigger weight loss. Spread over three meals (and a snack or two), you probably won't even notice the adjustment. Just remember your North Star. If your goal is to become healthier, focus less on counting calories and more on living your healthy life.

What Do I Eat?

Are you hungry yet? Let's talk about all the wonderful food you can eat on a veg-etarian keto diet. Before we get to the lists of what to love, limit, and lose (see the facing page), here are some general categories.

PLENTY OF GOOD FATS

A misconception about keto is that most fat comes from animal products; however, there are plenty of plant-based foods that have good fats in them. About 65 percent of your daily diet should come from healthy (unsaturated) fats, such as avocado, nuts, olive and coconut oils, whole-milk Greek yogurt, and eggs. Avoid trans fats, which are often found in foods such as frozen pizza, fast food, and French fries.

SOME (MOSTLY) PLANT-BASED PROTEINS

Hitting your 20 percent protein macro can be a little tough because many plant-based protein sources, such as beans and legumes, are high in carbs. How-ever, there are extraordinary sources of plant-based proteins that are also low in carbs, for example, spinach, mushrooms, and broccoli. Eggs are also an excep-tional source of low-carb protein if you choose to include them in your diet.

VERY FEW CARBS

The fewer carbs you consume, the faster you will reach (and maintain) ketosis. But not all carbs are the same. Complex carbohydrates, such as those found in vege-tables, take longer to digest and are a more stable source of energy than simple carbohydrates (e.g., table sugar).

Restricting your carb intake to about 15 percent takes some intentional choices (because certain fruits and vegetables are carb heavy), but there are plenty of low-carb options to choose from, such as spinach, radishes, and raspberries. Rest assured, the carbs you do consume from fruits and vegetables will be of a higher quality than refined carbs because they are full of micronutrients.

Everyone is different—some people can occasionally have higher-carb vege-tables such as onions, tomatoes, and pumpkin and stay in ketosis, whereas others can't. Try to keep an open mind. All the recipes in this cookbook were designed with your target macros in mind.

DON'T FORGET YOUR MICRONUTRIENTS

Micronutrients include minerals and vitamins, the small but mighty nutrients your body needs for immune function, blood clotting, and bone health. Key micronutrients include potassium, magnesium, and calcium, which are found in nutrient-dense foods such as yogurt, leafy greens, and nuts.

FOODS TO LOVE, LIMIT, AND LOSE

This easy table is a quick reference guide to help you learn which foods to enjoy, limit, and avoid on a vegetarian keto diet. Though it's not exhaustive, this list will help you make smart choices.

	LOVE	LIMIT	LOSE
VEGETABLES	Cruciferous vegetables (broccoli, Brussels sprouts, cauliflower); leafy greens (arugula, chard, lettuces); mushrooms	Carrots, celery, cucumbers, eggplant, green beans, onions, radishes	Artichokes, corn, parsnips, potatoes, pumpkin, yams
FRUITS	Avocado, coconut, olives	Berries, currants, tomatoes	Apples, bananas, grapes, watermelon
GRAINS & FLOURS	Coconut flour, flaxseed meal	Cocoa powder (unsweetened), nut flours	Cornmeal, oats, rice, rye, wheat
ANIMAL PROTEIN & DAIRY	Eggs, full-fat dairy (cheese, half-and-half, sour cream)	Low-fat and nonfat dairy	Animal proteins
NUTS, SEEDS & LEGUMES	Flaxseed, pecans, poppy seeds, sunflower seeds	Almonds, chia seeds, hazelnuts, hemp seeds, walnuts	Black-eyed peas, lentils, peanuts
FATS & OILS	Avocado oil, butter, coconut oil, olive oil	Corn oil, peanut oil	Vegetable shortening
SWEETENERS, CONDIMENTS & SEASONINGS	Horseradish, mayonnaise, mustard, sugar-free spice blends	Citrus juice, pesto, salsa	Coconut aminos, spice blends and sauces with sugar
BEVERAGES	Coffee, tea, unsweetened full-fat coconut milk, water	Almond milk, hard liquor, vegetable broth, wine	Beer, juice, soda

What Do I Need to Stock Up On?

Having a well-stocked kitchen is the first step to success. To properly kick off your new vegetarian keto lifestyle, stock up on the shelf-stable pantry ingredients that you will be using the most, as well as some basic kitchen tools to help you prep.

GO-TO PANTRY INGREDIENTS

There are some definite themes in vegetarian keto cuisine—vegetable-forward casseroles, soups of various textures, and medleys with roasted vegetables, to name a few. In this section, you will find a general list of the shelf-stable pantry items you'll see repeated in the recipes of this cookbook to make it easy for you to stock up. Some of the items may be unfamiliar to you; however, they are lifesavers in the vegetarian keto kitchen.

Almond milk: If you don't drink almond milk regularly, I recommend buying it in packs of four 8-ounce cartons to have on hand for sauces and desserts.

Apple cider vinegar: It's not just for salad dressing. Some keto enthusiasts swear by a sip of ACV per day to boost energy and stimulate weight loss.

Bruschetta, jarred: A tablespoon of prepared red pepper bruschetta added to your Fondue (page 87)? Why not? I reach for DeLallo tapenades and spreads because DeLallo is a family-owned business that has offered high-quality, shelf-stable foods since 1950.

Coconut milk: Always select cans of unsweetened and full-fat coconut milk. The fat rises to the top, so don't forget to shake the can before using.

Garlic: Many savory recipes in this cookbook use garlic. To save some prep time, you can buy already minced garlic or substitute my favorite ingredient, garlic paste. I recommend the brand Amore, a food company that specializes in all sorts of pastes. Keep their anchovy paste in mind when it's time to make Bagna Cauda Dip (page 113).

Green chiles: Buy them whole or diced in a can. Spoon some into your scrambled eggs. Pulse them in a food processor with cilantro, lime juice, and onion for a spectacular salsa verde. I love Rio Luna chiles, because they are organic and the company believes in sustainable farming practices.

Hot sauce: Even if you're not a huge fan of spicy food, a dash of hot sauce adds a layer of complexity to savory foods.

If you're making a fresh move to both vegetarian and keto, the adjustment may seem daunting. But there are some simple steps you can take to make the transition easier, and they all have something in common: intention.

Shop with purpose. Whether you shop for groceries online or brave the supermarket, maintain your focus. Create a shopping list before you arrive and try not to deviate. The shelves will tempt you with processed keto products. Stick to your list.

Meal plan and prep. When you prepare in advance for your meals and shop exclusively for those ingredients, you are less likely to deviate from vegetarian keto choices. Wash your fruits and vegetables as soon as you get home to speed up prep come mealtime.

Mind your portions. If the recipe you want to cook serves six and no one else is eating with you, scale the recipe back to the number of portions you're sure you'll consume that week.

Lean on quick options when you're busy. Quick meals, such as scrambled eggs, smoothies, and soups, are ideal for when you're short on time. Keeping a stock of healthy keto snacks such as Zucchini Chips (page 84) and Chili Chocolate Fat Bombs (page 92) will also help when you're between meals.

Be smart about eating out. Enjoying food out from time to time is fun and relaxing—and perfectly fine as long as you remember your North Star. Choose tomato soup, a meat-free salad, or even some queso with a side of vegetables.

Nutritional yeast: Wildly popular with vegetarians and vegans, nutritional yeast is sold in the spice section of the supermarket and contains vital micronutrients. It tastes cheesy even though it has no dairy included.

Spice blends: Southwest spice blends with cumin and chile pepper are great for Taco Slaw (page 38) and add a fun flavor boost to Ranch Dressing (page 116). Just make sure the blends are sugar-free.

Vegetable broth: You can make your own Vegetable Broth (page 108); however, so many vegetarian keto recipes feature it that you may run out, so keep a quart or two of boxed broth on hand, preferably a low-sodium variety.

To keep things beginner-friendly (and to save you some cabinet space), the recipes in this cookbook require only the basic kitchen essentials.

- Blender
- Box grater
- Food processor
- Measuring cups and spoons
- Muffin tin (12-cup)
- Parchment paper

You can skip the parchment paper and use nonstick cooking spray instead, but be aware that the spray can add a few extra calories. Parchment paper is sold in individual sheets (my preference), as well as in a roll, like aluminum foil.

An optional tool I recommend is a rasp or zester. A rasp is an inexpensive grater that is phenomenal for zesting citrus, pasting garlic and ginger, and dealing with basically anything you need to grate very tiny.

Just a Few More Questions . . .

The world of keto is wide and growing wider by the day. When I started exploring whether a ketogenic vegetarian lifestyle was right for me, I had far more questions than answers. The following represents my personal advice to help you prepare for what you might encounter on your own keto journey.

Q: How do I deal with the keto flu?

A: Keto flu, or carb flu, is your body's way of adjusting to macronutrient ratios that are higher in fat and lower in carbohydrates. As you lose the first bit of water weight, you may become dehydrated, resulting in fatigue, headaches, and sore muscles for the first week or so. You may be tempted to turn back to carbohydrates to cure the symptoms, but hydration is what you need. Double down on water, electrolytes, and healthy fats such as avocados and nuts throughout the day to maintain your blood sugar level and fortify your body with the nutrition it needs to push forward.

Q: **Can I exercise on this diet?**

A: Physical activity is generally advised; however, if you've never exercised, are under the care of a physician, or are taking medication, I highly recommend that you confer with a medical professional who can guide you regarding the recommended intensity and frequency of your workouts. Proper hydration is a critical component of any exercise regimen.

Q: **Should I add intermittent fasting?**

A: I regularly fast to maintain cellular health; however, if you are not used to fasting on a regular basis, a lack of food for extended periods coupled with this change in your diet may make you irritable. If there are people in your household who are not following the vegetarian keto diet, it may be difficult to resist other foods. Additionally, if you are underweight, pregnant, or nursing, your focus should be to consume sufficient calories throughout the day unless a qualified medical professional advises you otherwise.

Q: **Can I drink alcohol?**

A: Yes, in moderation. If your goal is fat loss, drinking alcohol will impede your progress. Spirits, such as whiskey and vodka, are preferable to beer and wine, but be careful of high-carb juices and premade mixers. Add lots of ice and pair spirits with soda water instead. Also note that when in ketosis, you'll likely feel the effects of alcohol more rapidly.

Q: **Do I need to take any supplements?**

A: If a medical professional has informed you that you are deficient in certain vitamins or minerals, alert them about your interest in a ketogenic vegetarian diet and follow their recommendation. Generally speaking, if you do not have any preexisting medical conditions, the nutrients offered in a well-balanced diet should be sufficient without the need for supplements.

Q: **Should I snack on keto?**

A: Once you reach ketosis, your hunger hormones will stabilize and your cravings between meals should subside. Until then, a daily snack or two from chapter 6 will help you ease into this new lifestyle. Taco Tots (page 88),

Parmesan Radishes (page 86), and Cookie Fat Bombs (page 91) are all great choices. When you're on the go, consider seaweed crisps, flaxseed tortilla chips, or a few nuts.

Q: **What about coffee and tea?**

A: Black coffee and tea are perfectly acceptable beverages. Unless otherwise specified, tea and coffee are caffeinated, which will increase your resting metabolic rate and can accelerate your heartbeat. Avoid adding sweeteners, if possible. If you like dairy in your coffee or tea, I recommend heavy cream or half-and-half, because milk is significantly higher in carbohydrates.

Meal Plan and Recipes

All that's left is to learn about some spectacular recipes and how you're going to easily fit their preparation into your routine. First, some details on the 14-day meal plan, then, some context about the recipes.

THE 14-DAY MEAL PLAN

This meal plan was made for one person: you! You'll have three nutritious meals per day. Although some of the recipes in this book are fun to dig into when you have some extra time, most of the recipes in the meal plan are designed with ease in mind: quick or make-ahead breakfasts, salads and sandwiches for lunch, and nourishing dinners that you can make in 45 minutes or less. Many of the recipes will give you leftovers, some of which are called for in the meal plan so you don't have to cook every meal from scratch. Recipes with leftovers that aren't accounted for in the plan will be marked with the portion size for one person—refer to the serving sizes for these dishes and decide if you'd prefer to divide the recipe. The recipes also use overlapping ingredients from one recipe to the next so you can spend less time shopping. If you'd like more information or recommendations on snacks, please refer to the Q&A on page 10 or see the recipes in chapter 6 (page 83).

THE RECIPES

Every recipe in this cookbook includes a full nutritional panel, macros, and serving sizes so you can be sure you are well nourished and eating the right amount. Most of the recipes include tips to make things easier—such as substitute ingredients, flavor variations, and even egg-free options. You'll also see the following dietary labels:

V   Vegan

DF   Dairy-Free (not included if the recipe is vegan)

EF   Egg-Free (not included if the recipe is vegan)

GF   Gluten-Free (When buying gluten-free products, always check the packaging to make sure the label specifies that the food was produced in a gluten-free facility.)

NF   Nut-Free

SF   Soy-Free

The following convenience labels will mark if a dish is:

Q   Quick (can be made in 30 minutes or less)

OP   One-Pot (only requires one piece of equipment to cook, such as a pot, skillet, or baking dish)

5   5-Ingredient (uses 5 or fewer ingredients, not including salt/pepper/oil/butter/ghee/water/cooking spray)

14-DAY MEAL PLAN

WEEK 1	BREAKFAST	LUNCH	DINNER
MONDAY	French Toast Egg Loaf (page 34)	Open-Faced Caprese Sandwich (page 48) (1 sandwich)	Egg Foo Young (page 79) (¼ recipe)
TUESDAY	Chocolate Mint Smoothie (page 26)	Egg White Salad (page 44)	Cream of Mushroom Soup (page 55)
WEDNESDAY	*French Toast Egg Loaf leftovers*	"B"LT (page 46)	Green Chile Stew (page 59)
THURSDAY	Cacao Crunch Cereal (page 27)	*Egg White Salad leftovers*	Green Bean and Mushroom Casserole (page 72)
FRIDAY	Blackberry Cheesecake Smoothie (page 25) (½ recipe)	*Green Chile Stew leftovers*	*Cream of Mushroom Soup leftovers*
SATURDAY	Hazelnut "Sausage" (page 29) and eggs (3 patties)	*Green Bean and Mushroom Casserole leftovers*	"Bacon" Spinach Salad (page 41) (½ recipe)
SUNDAY	Mushroom Feta Omelet (page 31)	Southwest Lettuce Cups (page 45) (½ recipe)	Shirataki Florentine (page 66) (½ recipe)

WEEK 1 SHOPPING LIST

To make your meal planning easier, here is a list of what you should buy for this week. But check your refrigerator and pantry before you go shopping; you may already have some of these items.

EGGS AND DAIRY

Butter (1 pound)

Cheese, feta, crumbled (4 ounces)

Cheese, fresh mozzarella (8 ounces)

Cheese, vegetarian Parmesan, grated (5 ounces) (The recipes in this book call for vegetarian Parmesan because Parmesan ordinarily contains animal rennet; always check the label.)

Cream cheese, full-fat (16 ounces)

Cream, heavy (16 ounces)

Eggs (4 dozen)

PRODUCE

Arugula (5 ounces)
Avocados (2)
Basil, fresh (1 bunch)
Bean sprouts (4 ounces)
Blackberries, fresh or frozen
    (6 ounces)
Butter lettuce (1 head)
Cabbage (1 head)
Carrots, large (2)
Cauliflower (1 head)
Celery (1 bunch)
Cilantro (1 bunch)
Garlic (1 head)
Ginger (1-inch knob)
Green beans (1 pound)
Italian parsley (1 bunch)

Jalapeño peppers (2)
Leeks (2)
Lemon (1)
Limes (2)
Mint (1 bunch)
Mushrooms (24 ounces)
Onion, white (1)
Onion, yellow (1)
Rosemary, fresh (1 bunch)
Scallions (1 bunch)
Shallots (5)
Spinach, baby (20 ounces)
Thyme (1 bunch)
Tomatoes, grape (10 ounces)
Tomatoes, Roma (4)
Zucchini, large (2)

OTHER

Almond milk (1 quart)
Shirataki noodles (7 ounces)

Tempeh (8 ounces)

PANTRY

Almond flour
Almonds, slivered
Baking powder
Bay leaf
Cacao nibs
Cayenne pepper
Chia seeds
Chiles, canned green
Chili powder
Cinnamon, ground
Coconut, shredded, unsweetened
Coconut milk, unsweetened, full-fat
Cumin, ground
Erythritol (brown)

Erythritol (regular)
Fennel seeds
Flour, hazelnut
Flour, oat
Garlic powder
Hot sauce
Maple syrup
Mayonnaise
MCT oil powder
Milk, nondairy
Mustard, Dijon
Nutmeg, ground
Oil, olive
Oil, extra-virgin olive

Oregano, dried

Parsley, dried

Paprika, smoked and sweet

Pecans

Pepper, black

Protein powder, sugar-free, soy-free
(both chocolate and vanilla
flavors)

Pumpkin seeds, shelled

Sage, ground

Salt

Soy sauce, gluten-free

Stevia, liquid

Sunflower seeds

Thyme, dried

Tomatoes, diced

Vegetable oil

Vinegar, balsamic

WEEK 1 PREP AHEAD

As you prepare for your first week of planned meals, there are some steps you can take in advance to make sure that you stay on track. Here are some things you can prep ahead to make the week easier.

SUNDAY

- Make the French Toast Egg Loaf, cool, and slice. Reserve one slice for breakfast on Monday and freeze the rest.
- Make the Basic Bread, cool, and slice. Reserve one slice for your Open-Faced Caprese Sandwich on Monday and freeze the rest.
- Prepare the batter for Egg Foo Young.

MONDAY

- Prepare the Pico de Gallo and hard-boil the eggs for Egg White Salad and "Bacon" Spinach Salad.
- Make a full batch of Vegetable Broth, cool, freeze into 1-cup portions, and thaw as needed during both weeks.
- Prepare the Cacao Crunch Cereal and divide into two servings—one for Thursday of this week, one for week 2.

TUESDAY

- Remove one slice of French Toast Egg Loaf from the freezer and thaw in the refrigerator for breakfast on Wednesday. Remove two slices of Basic Bread from the freezer and thaw in the refrigerator for your "B"LT on Wednesday.
- Prepare the Tempeh "Bacon" for your "B"LT and "Bacon" Spinach Salad.
- Prepare the Green Chile Stew through step 3, cool, and refrigerate.

FRIDAY

- Make the Balsamic Vinaigrette.
- Cook the Hazelnut "Sausage," cool, and refrigerate one serving for Saturday morning. Freeze the remaining servings.
- Roast the vegetables for Southwest Lettuce Cups.

WEEK 2	BREAKFAST	LUNCH	DINNER
MONDAY	Egg Muffins (page 30)	Taco Slaw (page 38) (½ recipe)	Garlic Fried Cauliflower Rice (page 78) (½ recipe)
TUESDAY	Morning Mocha Shake (page 24)	Roasted Vegetable Wrap (page 47) (1 wrap)	Southwest Lettuce Cups (page 45)
WEDNESDAY	Brussel Browns (page 28) and Bulletproof Coffee (page 23)	Southwest Lettuce Cups leftovers	Cayenne Pepper Vegetable Bake (page 73) (½ recipe)
THURSDAY	Egg Muffins leftovers	Garlic Fried Cauliflower Rice leftovers	Portabella Mushroom Margherita Pizza (page 69)
FRIDAY	Brussel Browns leftovers and Hot Almond Chocolate (page 22)	Cayenne Pepper Vegetable Bake leftovers	Chipotle Chili (page 60)
SATURDAY	Cacao Crunch Cereal leftovers (from week 1)	Joe's Keto Salad (page 42) (½ recipe)	Portabella Mushroom Pizza leftovers
SUNDAY	Egg Muffins leftovers	Chipotle Chili leftovers	Sesame Bok Choy Ramen (page 58) (½ recipe)

WEEK 2 SHOPPING LIST

Note: *This list does not include pantry or refrigerator staples that will carry over from week 1.*

EGGS AND DAIRY
Cheese, feta (2 ounces)
Cheese, shredded mozzarella (8 ounces)
Eggs (1 dozen)

PRODUCE
Asparagus (1 bunch)   Avocados, medium (3)

Baby bok choy (1 head)
Basil, fresh (1 bunch)
Bell pepper, any color, medium (1)
Brussels sprouts (32 ounces)
Cabbage (1 head)
Carrots, large (5)
Cauliflower (1 head)
Celery (1 head)
Cilantro (1 bunch)
Coleslaw mix (10 ounces)
Cucumber, English (1)
Garlic (1 head)
Ginger (2-inch knob)
Lemon (1)

Lettuce, Romaine hearts (2)
Mushroom, portabella (6 large)
Onion (1)
Parsley (1 bunch)
Radishes (1 bunch)
Scallions (2 bunches)
Shallot, medium (1)
Spinach (10 ounces)
Squash, yellow, small (1)
Tomatoes, grape (10 ounces)
Tomatoes, medium (4)
Turnips, medium (2)
Zucchini, small (3)

FROZEN
Cauliflower, riced (48 ounces)

Peas (10 ounces)

OTHER
Almond milk, unsweetened (1 quart)
Orange juice (8 ounces)
Shirataki noodles (7 ounces)

Soy crumbles (10 ounces)
Sprouted tofu (14 ounces)

PANTRY
Apple cider vinegar
Black olives, sliced
Chipotle peppers in adobo
Coconut milk, unsweetened, full-fat
Coffee
Ginger, ground
Marinara sauce
Mustard powder
Nonstick cooking spray
Nutritional yeast
Onion powder
Peanuts, chopped
Pimento peppers

Sesame oil
Taco seasoning
Tahini
Tamari
Tomato paste
Turmeric
Vegan Worcestershire sauce

WEEK 2 PREP AHEAD

By now, you're a pro at prepping. Here are some things you can make in advance as you gear up for week 2.

SUNDAY
- Prepare the Egg Muffins. Cool and refrigerate three servings—one for Monday, one for Thursday, and one for Sunday. Freeze the rest.
- Roast the vegetables for the Roasted Vegetable Wrap, Cayenne Pepper Vegetable Bake, and Southwest Lettuce Cups.
- Make the Avocado Goddess Dressing.

TUESDAY
- Prepare the Brussel Browns. Cool, reserve, and refrigerate two portions for Wednesday and Friday mornings. Freeze the rest.
- Make the salad dressing for Joe's Keto Salad and refrigerate.

THURSDAY
- Prepare the Chipotle Chili through step 2 to cook the vegetables. Refrigerate when done. On Friday night, pull out those precooked vegetables and move straight to step 3.

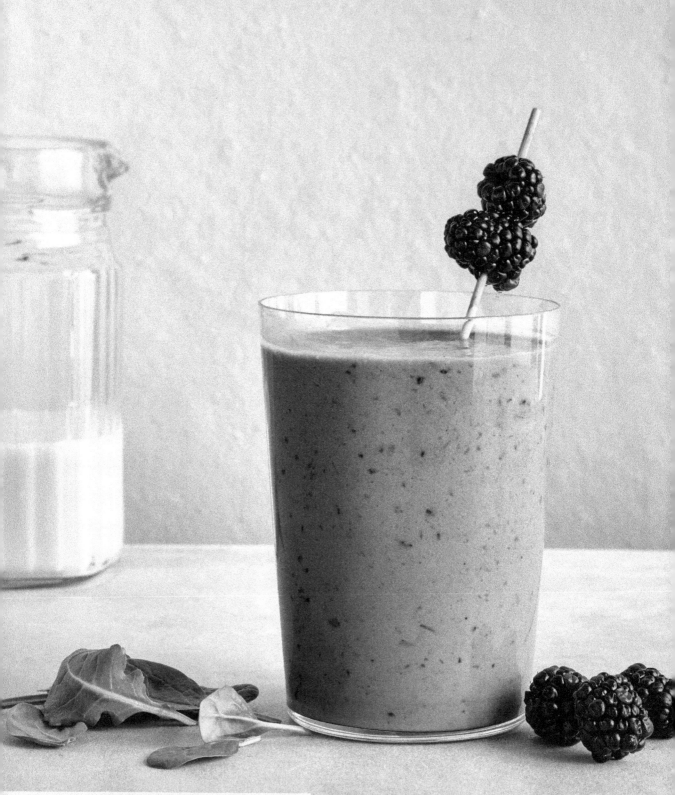
Blackberry Cheesecake Smoothie, page 25

CHAPTER 2

Breakfast and Beverages

Hot Almond Chocolate EF 5 GF OP Q SF 22

Bulletproof Coffee EF 5 GF NF OP Q SF 23

Morning Mocha Shake EF 5 GF OP Q SF 24

Blackberry Cheesecake Smoothie EF GF OP Q SF 25

Chocolate Mint Smoothie EF GF OP Q SF 26

Cacao Crunch Cereal GF OP Q SF V 27

Brussel Browns DF 5 GF NF Q SF 28

Hazelnut "Sausage" DF GF Q SF 29

Egg Muffins DF 5 GF Q SF 30

Mushroom Feta Omelet GF NF Q SF 31

Shakshuka GF NF OP SF 32

French Toast Egg Loaf 5 GF NF Q SF 34

OP

Q

SF

Hot Almond Chocolate

A mug of this hot chocolate is perfect for a weekend morning when you want to indulge but stay keto-true. I'm a bit of an extract eccentric and love to replace the almond extract with peppermint extract for a holiday-themed treat.

SERVES 1 • COOK TIME: 5 minutes

2 tablespoons unsweetened cocoa powder

1 cup milk, divided

2½ teaspoons liquid stevia

½ cup heavy cream

½ teaspoon almond extract

1 In a small saucepan over medium-low heat, whisk together the cocoa, ½ cup of milk, and the stevia until dissolved.

2 Increase the heat to medium, add the remaining ½ cup of milk and the cream and whisk occasionally until hot, about 5 minutes.

3 Stir in the almond extract and serve.

TIP: Although most extracts contain few to no calories and pack a major flavor punch, they do contain alcohol. If your lifestyle is alcohol-free, consider cold-pressed almond oil instead.

PER SERVING (ENTIRE RECIPE): Calories: 585; Total fat: 52g; Protein: 13g; Total carbs: 22g; Fiber: 4g; Net carbs: 18g

MACROS: Fat: 80%; Protein: 9%; Carbs: 11%

VEGETARIAN KETOGENIC COOKBOOK FOR BEGINNERS

Bulletproof Coffee

Bulletproof coffee is a staple beverage in many keto diets, though you may be surprised by the ingredient list—butter and oil in coffee? The added fat and caffeine keep you full and energized long after you finish your cup.

EF

5

GF

NF

OP

Q

SF

SERVES 1 • PREP TIME: 5 minutes

1½ cups hot coffee

2 tablespoons MCT
  oil powder

2 tablespoons butter or ghee

1 Pour the hot coffee into a blender. Add the oil powder and butter. Blend until thoroughly mixed and frothy.

2 Pour into a large mug and enjoy.

RAW EGG VARIATION

To add protein, replace the MCT oil powder with 1 raw egg. It may sound strange, but the egg adds an appealing creamy texture, and although the hot coffee cooks the egg, there will be no hint of cooked proteins.

PROTEIN POWDER VARIATION

You could also add a scoop or two of protein powder.

SPICED VARIATION

Add 1 teaspoon of ground cinnamon and a little keto-friendly sweetener to your bulletproof mixture for a delicious spiced version.

TIP: If you're new to the keto diet, you will want to start slow with MCT oil powder. It is powerful, so work your way up to 2 tablespoons over the course of a few weeks.

PER SERVING (ENTIRE RECIPE): Calories: 463; Total fat: 51g; Protein: 1g; Total carbs: 0g; Fiber: 0g; Net carbs: 0g

MACROS: Fat: 99%; Protein: 1%; Carbs: 0%

Morning Mocha Shake

Protein powder is a very convenient shortcut for healthy breakfasts and a timesaver for busy mornings; however, many protein powders have additives such as maltodextrin, which can cause gastrointestinal distress. Always read nutrition labels carefully.

SERVES 1 • PREP TIME: 5 minutes

6 frozen coconut milk cubes (see tip)

½ cup brewed coffee

3 tablespoons sugar-free, soy-free chocolate protein powder

In a blender, combine all the ingredients and blend until smooth. Serve immediately.

TIP: Coconut milk freezes beautifully. Shake the can well and distribute it evenly into an ice cube tray. Each frozen coconut cube will be about 3 tablespoons.

PER SERVING (ENTIRE RECIPE): Calories: 580; Total fat: 50g; Protein: 24g; Total carbs: 16g; Fiber: 4g; Net carbs: 12g

MACROS: Fat: 77%; Protein: 16%; Carbs: 7%

Blackberry Cheesecake Smoothie

EF

GF

OP

Q

SF

Though you should limit your berry consumption on the keto diet, black-berries are extremely rich in fiber (about 5 grams in ⅔ cup) as well as vitamins C and K. Blackberry seeds are also a good source of protein, omega-3 fatty acids, and fiber, so don't strain this smoothie after blending.

SERVES 2 • PREP TIME: 10 minutes

1 cup unsweetened
   almond milk

⅔ cup full-fat cream cheese

½ cup fresh or frozen
   blackberries

½ cup shredded fresh
   baby spinach

1 scoop sugar-free, soy-free
   vanilla protein powder

1 tablespoon erythritol

1 In a blender, combine all the ingredients and blend until smooth.

2 Pour into two glasses and serve immediately.

TIP: This is not an overly sweet smoothie. The black-berries add a certain tartness, so drinking a large amount won't be overwhelming. You could use this entire recipe as one serving and enjoy a quick 754-calorie meal.

PER SERVING (½ RECIPE): Calories: 377; Total fat: 29g; Protein: 19g; Total carbs: 10g; Fiber: 5g; Net carbs: 5g

MACROS: Fat: 70%; Protein: 10%; Carbs: 20%

Chocolate Mint Smoothie

Avocado adds a luscious richness to just about every dish, especially this breakfast smoothie. Though you can substitute any milk you prefer, I particularly like how almond milk mellows the characteristic flavor of the spinach in this recipe, which allows the chocolate and mint to take center stage.

SERVES 1 • PREP TIME: 5 minutes

½ cup fresh spinach

½ cup almond milk

½ cup water

½ ripe avocado, pitted and peeled

2 tablespoons sugar-free, soy-free chocolate protein powder

1 tablespoon minced fresh mint

1 tablespoon erythritol

3 ice cubes

In a blender, combine all the ingredients and blend until smooth. Serve immediately.

TIP: To ensure this smoothie is vegan, select a plant-based protein powder.

PER SERVING (ENTIRE RECIPE): Calories: 225; Total fat: 14g; Protein: 17g; Total carbs: 22g; Fiber: 7g; Net carbs: 15g

MACROS: Fat: 56%; Protein: 25%; Carbs: 19%

Cacao Crunch Cereal

Craving cereal without all the sugar? This healthy combination will give you that crunch and sweetness alongside a generous dose of fiber and healthy fats. Feel free to add erythritol or a couple of berries for natural sweetness. Strawberries and cacao nibs are a delicious combination.

GF
OP
Q
SF
V

SERVES 2 • PREP TIME: 5 minutes

½ cup slivered almonds

2 tablespoons unsweet-
ened shredded or
flaked coconut

2 tablespoons chia seeds

2 tablespoons cacao nibs

2 tablespoons sun-
flower seeds

Unsweetened nondairy milk
of choice, for serving

1 In a small bowl, combine the almonds, coconut, chia seeds, cacao nibs, and sunflower seeds. Divide into two bowls.

2 Pour in the nondairy milk and serve.

PER SERVING (½ RECIPE, CEREAL ONLY): Calories: 325; Total fat: 27; Protein: 10g; Total carbs: 17g; Fiber: 12g; Net carbs: 5g

MACROS: Fat: 70%; Protein: 11%; Carbs: 19%

Brussel Browns

Traditional hash browns are made with potatoes and other root vege-
tables, which are high in carbohydrates and not keto-friendly. Brussel
browns feature Brussels sprouts instead, which pair wonderfully with
eggs and freeze beautifully. In a pinch, Brussel browns can also substitute
for bread in a keto egg sandwich.

SERVES 4 • PREP TIME: 5 minutes **• COOK TIME:** 5 minutes

2 large eggs

½ teaspoon garlic powder

½ teaspoon salt

½ teaspoon freshly ground
black pepper

2 cups shredded
Brussels sprouts

1 shallot, thinly sliced

1 tablespoon vegetable oil

1 In a large bowl, whisk together the eggs, garlic
powder, salt, and pepper. Add the Brussels sprouts
and shallot and toss to combine.

2 In a large skillet over medium-high heat, heat the
oil until shimmering. Divide the Brussels sprout
mixture into four piles in the pan and press with a
spatula to flatten them.

3 Cook until golden and crisp, about 3 minutes
per side.

TIP: If you purchase already-shredded Brussels
sprouts, give them a quick chop so your piles com-
press more easily. This will also ensure they cook
evenly and the edges don't burn.

PER SERVING (1 BRUSSEL BROWN): Calories: 125;
Total fat: 8g; Protein: 5g; Total carbs: 9g; Fiber: 2g;
Net carbs: 7g

MACROS: Fat: 58%; Protein: 16%; Carbs: 26%

Hazelnut "Sausage"

DF
GF
Q
SF

If you're new to a vegetarian lifestyle, you might be searching for a familiar protein to enjoy with your eggs in the morning. How about a breakfast sausage . . . that isn't really sausage? This recipe mimics both the texture and the flavor of sausage, so you won't feel like you're missing out.

MAKES 9 PATTIES • PREP TIME: 10 minutes **• COOK TIME:** 15 minutes

2 large eggs

½ cup hazelnut flour

1¼ cups oat flour

1½ teaspoons liquid stevia

1 teaspoon brown erythritol

1 teaspoon salt

½ teaspoon dried sage

½ teaspoon dried thyme

⅛ teaspoon grated nutmeg

Freshly ground black pepper

1 teaspoon fennel seeds

½ cup vegetable oil

1   In a food processor, combine the eggs, hazelnut and oat flours, stevia, erythritol, salt, sage, thyme, nutmeg, and pepper. Pulse until the mixture forms a thick paste. Add the fennel seeds and pulse lightly to incorporate, keeping the seeds intact.

2   Form the mixture into 9 patties, about 2½ tablespoons each.

3   In a large pan over medium-high heat, heat the oil until shimmering. Carefully drop the patties into the pan (working in batches if necessary), spacing them 1 inch apart. Cook for about 4 minutes per side until golden brown.

4   Drain the patties on a paper towel–lined plate or wire rack.

TIP: If you are unable to find hazelnut flour, pulverize whole hazelnuts in a blender or food processor until they reach a powdered consistency (don't blend too much or you'll have nut butter). Alternatively, try almond flour.

PER SERVING (3 PATTIES): Calories: 697; Total fat: 54g; Protein: 14g; Total carbs: 42g; Fiber: 9g; Net carbs: 33g

MACROS: Fat: 70%; Protein: 8%; Carbs: 22%

Egg Muffins

When it comes to egg muffins, I've experimented with a variety of flavor combos, but I always come back to this spinach and asparagus dynamic duo. These muffins make for a handheld, fiber-rich breakfast that is packed with protein.

MAKES 12 MUFFINS • PREP TIME: 5 minutes • COOK TIME: 20 minutes

Nonstick cooking spray

8 large eggs

¼ cup almond milk

1 cup chopped fresh spinach

1 cup finely chopped asparagus, tough ends discarded

½ teaspoon salt

½ teaspoon onion powder

½ teaspoon freshly
ground pepper

1 Preheat the oven to 350°F. Grease a 12-cup muffin pan with cooking spray.

2 In a large bowl, whisk the eggs until beaten. Add the almond milk and whisk to combine. Add the spinach, asparagus, salt, onion powder, and pepper and whisk until well mixed.

3 Divide the egg mixture evenly between the cups of the muffin pan.

4 Bake for 20 minutes or until the egg is set. Cool for 5 minutes before serving hot, or cool completely and refrigerate the muffins in an airtight container for up to 1 week.

TIP: Leftover muffins are a great ready-made breakfast. To reheat, microwave one muffin for about 30 seconds and enjoy.

PER SERVING (1 EGG MUFFIN): Calories: 56; Total fat: 4g; Protein: 5g; Total carbs: 1g; Fiber: <1g; Net carbs: <1g

MACROS: Fat: 64%; Protein: 36%; Carbs: <1%

Mushroom Feta Omelet

It'll be tempting to flip your mushrooms as they cook in this omelet, but try to leave them be. Allowing them to remain undisturbed as they cook allows them to achieve a nice sear, which deepens their flavor.

SERVES 1 • PREP TIME: 5 minutes **• COOK TIME:** 15 minutes

2 tablespoons olive oil, divided

1 tablespoon minced shallot

1 cup sliced mushrooms

3 large eggs

1 tablespoon heavy cream

1 teaspoon dried parsley

¼ teaspoon salt

¼ teaspoon freshly ground black pepper

2 tablespoons crumbled feta

1. In a large skillet over medium heat, heat 1 tablespoon of olive oil until shimmering. Add the shallot and cook for 2 minutes, stirring occasionally, until fragrant. Add the mushrooms and cook, undisturbed, for 5 minutes, until softened. Transfer the mushroom mixture to a plate.

2. In a medium bowl, combine the eggs, cream, parsley, salt, and pepper. Whisk until well mixed.

3. Add the remaining 1 tablespoon of oil to the skillet and pour in the egg mixture. Cook until the edges are brown and the egg is set, about 5 minutes.

4. Place the mushrooms on one half of the omelet. Sprinkle the feta over the mushrooms.

5. Fold the omelet in half, sandwiching the mushrooms and cheese in the middle, and serve.

TIP: You can also use dried mushrooms in this recipe—just soak them in warm water or vegetable stock until rehydrated before adding to the skillet. You can even drink the leftover mushroom broth, which boosts liver health. Be sure to strain any sediment from the bowl before consuming.

PER SERVING (1 OMELET): Calories: 596; Total fat: 53g; Protein: 25g; Total carbs: 7g; Fiber: 1g; Net carbs: 6g

MACROS: Fat: 80%; Protein: 17%; Carbs: 3%

Shakshuka

Shakshuka, or eggs baked in a spicy tomato-based sauce, is common in both North African and Israeli cuisine. This recipe features an olive oil–tomato base to keep ratios favorable for a ketogenic approach, and it adds spinach for an extra boost of nutrition. Adjust the spices to your liking, omitting the red pepper flakes entirely if you prefer things less spicy.

SERVES 4 • PREP TIME: 10 minutes **• COOK TIME:** 30 minutes

½ cup plus 2 tablespoons olive oil, divided

½ small yellow onion, finely diced

1 red bell pepper, finely diced

1 (14-ounce) can crushed tomatoes, with juices

6 ounces frozen spinach, thawed and drained (about 1½ cups)

2 cloves garlic, finely minced

1 tablespoon coarsely chopped capers

1 to 2 teaspoons red pepper flakes (optional)

1 teaspoon smoked paprika

6 large eggs

¼ teaspoon freshly ground black pepper

¾ cup crumbled feta or goat cheese

¼ cup chopped fresh flat-leaf parsley or cilantro

1 Preheat the oven to broil.

2 In a medium, deep, oven-safe skillet over medium-high heat, heat 1 tablespoon olive oil until shimmering. Add the onion and bell pepper and sauté until softened, 5 to 8 minutes.

3 Add the crushed tomatoes and their juices, ½ cup of olive oil, spinach, garlic, capers, red pepper flakes (if using), and paprika, stirring to combine. Bring to a boil, then reduce the heat to low. Cover and simmer for 5 minutes.

4 Uncover the skillet and use a spoon to make 6 wells in the sauce. Gently crack an egg into each well, being careful not to let the eggs touch. Add the black pepper, then cover and cook until the yolks are just set, 8 to 10 minutes. Eight minutes will yield softer yolks, whereas 10 minutes will yield firmer yolks.

5 Uncover the skillet and spread the crumbled cheese over the eggs and sauce. Transfer to the oven and broil until the cheese is just slightly browned and bubbly, 3 to 5 minutes. Drizzle with the remaining 1 tablespoon olive oil, top with the chopped parsley, and serve warm.

TIP: For even faster preparation, substitute 1 jar of low-carb, no-sugar-added marinara sauce for the onion, bell pepper, crushed tomatoes, and garlic. Skip steps 2 and 3, season the marinara sauce with paprika and red pepper flakes, and bring to a simmer before cracking in the eggs.

PER SERVING (¼ RECIPE): Calories: 476, Total fat: 40g, Protein: 17g; Total carbs: 12g, Fiber: 5g, Net carbs: 7g

MACROS: Fat: 76%; Protein: 14%; Carbs: 10%

French Toast Egg Loaf

Egg loaves like this one are a breakfast canvas, just waiting for your brushstrokes. Experiment with savory preparations, too. Instead of cinnamon, try sprinkling in some diced chives or roasted red peppers.

MAKES 12 SLICES • PREP TIME: 5 minutes • COOK TIME: 25 minutes

8 tablespoons (1 stick) butter, at room temperature, plus more for greasing

8 ounces cream cheese, at room temperature

8 large eggs

1 teaspoon ground cinnamon

1 teaspoon erythritol

1 Preheat the oven to 350°F. Grease a 9-by-5-inch loaf pan with butter.

2 In a blender, combine all the ingredients and blend until completely smooth. Pour the batter into the prepared pan.

3 Bake for 25 minutes or until a toothpick inserted into the center of the loaf comes out clean.

TIP: Salted butter will offer you a balanced egg loaf, whereas unsalted butter will bring the cinnamon a bit more to the forefront.

PER SERVING (1 SLICE): Calories: 186; Total fat: 18g; Protein: 5g; Total carbs: 2g; Fiber: <1g; Net carbs: 2g

MACROS: Fat: 87%; Protein: 11%; Carbs: 2%

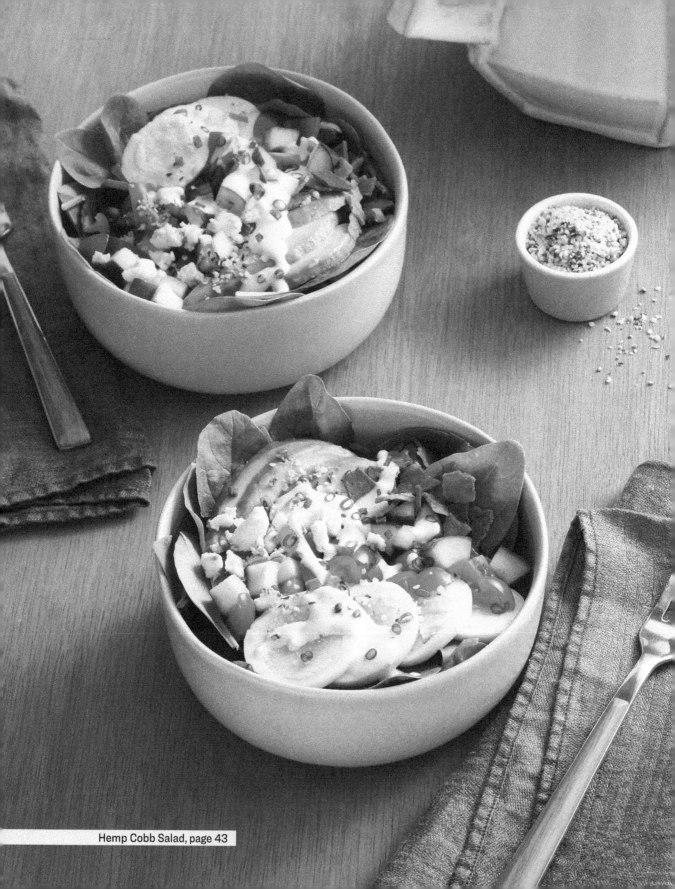

Hemp Cobb Salad, page 43

CHAPTER 3

Salads and Sandwiches

Taco Slaw DF GF NF Q 38

Ranch Broccoli Slaw 5 GF OP Q SF 39

Buon Gusto Salad GF NF Q 40

"Bacon" Spinach Salad DF GF NF OP Q 41

Joe's Keto Salad Q SF 42

Hemp Cobb Salad GF NF Q 43

Egg White Salad DF 5 GF NF Q SF 44

Southwest Lettuce Cups DF GF Q SF 45

"B"LT 5 GF NF OP Q 46

Roasted Vegetable Wrap GF NF Q SF V 47

Open-Faced Caprese Sandwich GF Q SF 48

DF
GF
NF
Q

Taco Slaw

Nothing says "fiesta" like tacos, but the carbohydrates in the tortillas are sure to take you out of ketosis. When the taco cravings hit, this taco slaw is just what you need. For some extra smokiness, toast the pumpkin seeds in a dry pan over medium heat for two to three minutes until they're fragrant, stirring frequently so they don't burn.

SERVES 2 • PREP TIME: 10 minutes, plus 15 minutes to rest • **COOK TIME:** 10 minutes

1 cup soy crumbles

2 teaspoons taco seasoning, divided

1 (10-ounce) bag coleslaw mix or shredded cabbage

½ teaspoon salt, plus more for seasoning

2 scallions, thinly sliced, white and green parts

½ cup grated carrot

¼ cup chopped fresh cilantro

3 tablespoons mayonnaise

2 tablespoons freshly squeezed orange juice

1 tablespoon pickled jalapeño brine (see tip)

Freshly ground black pepper

3 tablespoons toasted pumpkin seeds

1. Season the soy crumbles with 1 teaspoon of taco seasoning and cook according to the package instructions.

2. In a medium bowl, toss the coleslaw with the salt and let it sit for about 15 minutes. Drain any excess liquid that accumulates in the bottom of the bowl.

3. To the coleslaw, add the scallions, carrot, and cilantro and toss.

4. In a small bowl, combine the mayonnaise, orange juice, brine, and remaining 1 teaspoon taco seasoning and pour the dressing over the slaw mixture. Toss the slaw and season with salt and pepper.

5. Arrange the slaw on plates. Top with the soy crumbles and garnish with the pumpkin seeds.

TIP: The brine in jarred pickles and jalapeños is a flavor bomb waiting to explode. Substitute brine for recipes that call for vinegar—just strain out the peppercorns and seeds, which may overpower your dish.

PER SERVING (½ RECIPE): Calories: 343; Total fat: 22g; Protein: 19g; Total carbs: 28g; Fiber: 9g; Net carbs: 19g

MACROS: Fat: 58%; Protein: 22%; Carbs: 20%

Ranch Broccoli Slaw

5

GF

OP

Q

SF

Shredded broccoli slaw is available in most grocery stores; however, 1 ½ cups of grated or finely chopped broccoli works just as well for this salad. One cup of broccoli slaw provides 50 percent of the recommended daily value for vitamin A and is a naturally filling source of fiber. With a half cup of almonds per serving, your macros will be perfectly aligned for ketosis.

SERVES 2 • PREP TIME: 5 minutes

1 (12-ounce) bag shredded broccoli slaw

1 cup sliced almonds

3 servings Ranch Dressing (page 116) or store-bought ranch dressing

½ cup sliced radishes

¼ cup dried sugar-free cranberries

In a large bowl, combine all the ingredients and toss to coat. Serve immediately.

TIP: If you have any plain broccoli left over, toss it in 1 or 2 tablespoons of Bagna Cauda Dip (page 113) and roast for 20 minutes at 400° F for a comforting side dish.

PER SERVING (½ RECIPE): Calories: 546; Total fat: 35g; Protein: 20g; Total carbs: 42g; Fiber: 14g; Net carbs: 28g

MACROS: Fat: 58%; Protein: 15%; Carbs: 27%

Buon Gusto Salad

Buon gusto *is an Italian expression that means "good taste," and this salad fits that bill. Featuring many of the flavors you'd find in an Italian deli, this salad delivers all the antipasto without the extra carbs (or the meat, of course). If you prefer, replace the lettuce mix with one head of radicchio and one head of romaine lettuce.*

SERVES 2 • PREP TIME: 10 minutes

1 (10-ounce) bag Italian lettuce mix

½ cup sliced grape tomatoes

4 ounces vegan pepperoni

½ cup artichoke hearts, quartered

¼ cup Italian green olives, pitted

4 pepperoncini peppers, sliced

¼ cup shredded vegetarian Parmesan

3 tablespoons mayonnaise

2 tablespoons balsamic vinegar

1 tablespoon freshly ground black pepper

1 In a large bowl, combine the lettuce, tomatoes, pepperoni, artichoke hearts, olives, peppers, and Parmesan and toss well.

2 In a small bowl, combine the mayonnaise and balsamic vinegar. Pour the dressing over the salad and toss again. Season with the black pepper.

TIP: Vegan pepperoni can easily be omitted for those with soy allergies.

PER SERVING (½ RECIPE): Calories: 420; Total fat: 31g; Protein: 15g; Total carbs: 27g; Fiber: 14g; Net carbs: 13g

MACROS: Fat: 66%; Protein: 14%; Carbs: 20%

"Bacon" Spinach Salad

DF

GF

NF

OP

Q

Spinach is nature's boost for healthy blood, due to its high levels of iron and vitamin K. Like most dark, leafy vegetables, spinach is loaded with antioxidants, which are known to reduce inflammation, fight wrinkles, and give your skin a healthy glow.

SERVES 2 • PREP TIME: 5 minutes

1 (10-ounce) package
  baby spinach

4 slices Tempeh "Bacon"
  (page 119), crumbled

4 hard-boiled eggs, sliced

½ cup sliced mushrooms

2 tablespoons diced shallot

2 tablespoons Balsamic
  Vinaigrette (page 114) or
  store-bought balsamic
  vinaigrette

1 Scatter the spinach over a large dinner plate or platter.

2 Arrange the "bacon," eggs, mushrooms, and shallot on top of the spinach.

3 Drizzle with the Balsamic Vinaigrette and serve.

TIP: If you choose fresh spinach that isn't prewashed, remove the stems and swish the leaves around in cold water to ensure any bits of debris and dirt sink to the bottom. Pull the leaves out after 1 to 2 minutes and dry them well before serving. No one likes a soggy salad.

PER SERVING (½ RECIPE): Calories: 366; Total fat: 21g; Protein: 27g; Total carbs: 22g; Fiber: 4g; Net carbs: 18g

MACROS: Fat: 52%; Protein: 30%: Carbs: 18%

Joe's Keto Salad

Crafted in honor of Joe's Seafood, Prime Steak & Stone Crab in Las Vegas, this salad is the ideal blend of salty, fresh, and sweet. For an extra pop of flavor, the dressing infuses some of the ingredients found in Joe's mustard sauce.

SERVES 2 • PREP TIME: 10 minutes

FOR THE DRESSING

2 tablespoons minced
    pimento peppers

2 tablespoons mayonnaise

1 tablespoon apple
    cider vinegar

1 teaspoon mustard powder

1 teaspoon brown erythritol

1 teaspoon vegan
    Worcestershire

½ teaspoon erythritol

¼ teaspoon salt

FOR THE SALAD

2 romaine hearts,
    sliced thinly

8 grape tomatoes, halved

4 hard-boiled eggs, chopped

½ cup peeled, diced English
    cucumber

½ cup shredded carrot

2 tablespoons sliced
    black olives

2 tablespoons feta cheese

2 tablespoons peanuts

TO MAKE THE DRESSING

In a blender or food processor, combine all the dressing ingredients. Blend until smooth.

TO MAKE THE SALAD

In a large bowl, combine the romaine, tomatoes, eggs, cucumber, carrot, and olives. Cover with the dressing and toss to coat. Top with the feta and peanuts and serve immediately.

TIP: Experiment with different varieties of lettuce. Red leaf lettuce is a great substitute.

PER SERVING (½ RECIPE): Calories: 365; Total fat: 28g; Protein: 17g; Total carbs: 15g; Fiber: 5g; Net carbs: 10g

MACROS: Fat: 69%; Protein: 19%; Carbs: 12%

Hemp Cobb Salad

Cobb salads are a staple for keto eaters, and in this rendition, you'll get your salty crunch from vegan bacon. This super fresh, vegetable-loaded salad can be easily prepared in just a few minutes.

SERVES 2 • PREP TIME: 10 minutes

2 cups fresh spinach leaves

4 hard-boiled eggs, peeled and chopped

4 slices Tempeh "Bacon" (page 119), crumbled

1 avocado, pitted, peeled, and sliced

¼ cup diced tomato

¼ cup diced cucumber

4 tablespoons hemp seeds

2 tablespoons diced scallions, white and green parts

½ cup blue cheese crumbles

4 tablespoons Ranch Dressing (page 116) or store-bought ranch dressing

1 Divide the spinach leaves into two bowls.

2 Arrange half the eggs, "bacon," avocado, tomato, and cucumber in sections on top of each bowl of spinach.

3 Sprinkle each salad with half the hemp seeds, scallions, and blue cheese.

4 Top each salad with dressing and serve.

TIP: To store this salad for future use, prepare the ingredients and keep them in separate containers in the refrigerator for up to 3 days.

TIP: Follow Your Heart makes a killer bottled vegan ranch dressing that you can use in a pinch. And did you know McCormick Imitation Bacon Bits are vegan? Use either of these in place of the homemade staples in this recipe.

PER SERVING (½ RECIPE): Calories: 858; Total fat: 72g; Protein: 32g; Total carbs: 20g; Fiber: 9g; Net carbs: 11g

MACROS: Fat: 76%; Protein: 15%; Carbs: 9%

Egg White Salad

Trader Joe's delicious Spicy Ranchero Egg White Salad was my go-to keto lunch when I lived and worked in the Bay Area. I realized I could re-create it far more affordably at home, without the soy protein additives. To stay heart healthy, this recipe leaves out the egg yolks—it still delivers all the egg flavor, but none of the cholesterol.

SERVES 2 • PREP TIME: 10 minutes • **COOK TIME:** 15 minutes, plus 5 minutes to chill

8 large eggs

2 tablespoons mayonnaise

½ teaspoon salt

4 tablespoons Pico de Gallo (page 111) or store-bought pico de gallo, divided

1 Without cracking them, place the eggs in a medium pot and fill with enough cold water to cover them by 1 inch. Set over high heat and bring to a boil.

2 Remove from the heat and cover with a lid. Let stand for 14 minutes. During this time, fill a large bowl with ice water.

3 Transfer the eggs to the ice bath and let sit for 5 minutes. Peel the eggs, then slice them in half lengthwise and separate the yolks and whites. (Store the yolks in a resealable food container and snack on them during the week when you need a protein boost.)

4 In a small food processor, combine the egg whites, mayonnaise, and salt and pulse to your desired texture. Alternatively, mash by hand with a fork.

5 Transfer the mixture to a bowl and add 3 tablespoons of Pico de Gallo. Mix well.

6 Divide into two portions and top with the remaining Pico de Gallo.

TIP: Instant Pots make perfect hard-boiled eggs. Pour 1 cup of water into the pot and insert the trivet. Place the raw eggs on the trivet and lock the lid. Cook on high pressure for 5 minutes, allow the pressure to release naturally for 5 minutes, then carefully cool the eggs in an ice bath for 5 minutes before peeling.

PER SERVING (½ RECIPE): Calories: 407; Total fat: 32g; Protein: 25g; Total carbs: 3g; Fiber: <1g; Net carbs: <3g

MACROS: Fat: 71%; Protein: 24%; Carbs: 5%

Southwest Lettuce Cups

DF

GF

Q

SF

Lettuce wraps with Asian flavors took the world by storm several years ago; however, they are often very high in sodium and other unhealthy additives. This festive, Southwestern version offers a combination of roasted and fresh vegetables, with a pecan crunch. By dicing the vegetables before they roast, you're accelerating their cooking time.

SERVES 2 • PREP TIME: 5 minutes • **COOK TIME:** 25 minutes

1 cup diced zucchini

1 cup diced cauliflower

1 tablespoon olive oil

½ teaspoon paprika

½ teaspoon ground cumin

½ teaspoon garlic powder

½ teaspoon chili powder

¼ teaspoon salt

¼ teaspoon freshly ground
    black pepper

1 cup finely chopped pecans

2 tablespoons mayonnaise

1 tablespoon sriracha or a
    few dashes of hot sauce

⅓ cup grated cabbage

4 butter lettuce leaves

2 scallions, thinly sliced,
    white and green parts

1 Preheat the oven to 400°F. Line a baking sheet with parchment paper.

2 On the baking sheet, toss the zucchini and cauliflower with the olive oil, paprika, cumin, garlic powder, chili powder, salt, and pepper. Roast for 20 to 25 minutes, until tender.

3 Carefully transfer the vegetables to a medium bowl to cool for 5 minutes, then add the pecans and toss.

4 In a small bowl, combine the mayonnaise and sriracha. Add the cabbage and toss to coat.

5 Fill the lettuce leaves evenly with roasted vegetables and top with spicy cabbage and a sprinkle of scallions.

TIP: If you're eating with meat lovers, sauté some ground beef in a separate pan, seasoned with the same spices as your vegetables, for an inclusive experience for all.

PER SERVING (½ RECIPE): Calories: 584; Total fat: 57g; Protein: 8g; Total carbs: 18g; Fiber: 9g; Net carbs: 9g

MACROS: Fat: 88%; Protein: 5%; Carbs: 7%

"B"LT

Remaining successful on a vegetarian keto diet is infinitely easier when you have an arsenal of ultra-quick meals that come together in a flash. If you thought that some of your go-to, carb-rich favorites were off the table, think again. This "B"LT takes advantage of two homemade staples that are a match made in keto heaven.

SERVES 1 • PREP TIME: 5 minutes

2 tablespoons mayonnaise

2 slices Basic Bread
(page 117)

5 grape tomatoes, sliced

¼ teaspoon salt

2 butter lettuce leaves

2 slices Tempeh "Bacon"
(page 119)

1 Spread 1 tablespoon of mayonnaise on each slice of bread.

2 Top one slice of bread with the tomatoes, salt, lettuce, and "bacon" and place the second piece of bread on top.

TIP: Grape tomatoes contain 50 percent less carbohydrates than cherry tomatoes and are rich in vitamin C. Because they are consistent in size, it's a breeze to portion them out.

PER SERVING (1 SANDWICH): Calories: 666; Total fat: 57g; Protein: 24g; Total carbs: 22g; Fiber: 5g; Net carbs: 17g

MACROS: Fat: 77%; Protein: 14%; Carbs: 9%

Roasted Vegetable Wrap

Meet stuffed cabbage's sassy twin. Portable and lunchable, a wrap is a great way to pack in the nutrients you need to keep your energy up throughout the day. Out of Avocado Goddess Dressing (page 115)? Ranch Dressing (page 116) is a perfect understudy.

SERVES 2 • PREP TIME: 10 minutes • **COOK TIME:** 20 minutes

1 small yellow squash, diced

1 small zucchini, diced

2 tablespoons olive oil

½ teaspoon garlic powder

2 tablespoons minced pimento peppers

2 tablespoons Avocado Goddess Dressing (page 115) or store-bought green goddess dressing

4 cups water

1 teaspoon salt

2 large cabbage leaves

1 Preheat the oven to 400°F. Line a baking sheet with parchment paper.

2 On the baking sheet, toss the yellow squash and zucchini with the olive oil and garlic powder. Roast until tender, about 20 minutes.

3 Allow the roasted vegetables to cool for 5 to 10 minutes, then mix them in a medium bowl with the pimentos and avocado goddess dressing. Set aside.

4 Fill a large pot with 4 cups of water and bring to a boil over high heat. Add the salt and stir until dissolved.

5 Place the cabbage leaves in the boiling water for about 15 seconds, until they become pliable, then gently remove them with a pair of tongs. Pat the leaves dry.

6 Spread each cabbage leaf on a plate and top evenly with the vegetable mixture.

7 One at a time, fold the bottom of the leaf over the vegetables, fold over the sides, and roll forward (like you would a burrito). Serve immediately.

TIP: Just about any large, sturdy leaf will do to wrap your vegetables. Also try chard or collards, depending on what's freshest.

PER SERVING (1 WRAP): Calories: 183; Total fat: 17g; Protein: 2g; Total carbs: 8g; Fiber: 3g; Net carbs: 5g

MACROS: Fat: 84%; Protein: 4%; Carbs: 12%

Open-Faced Caprese Sandwich

This sandwich honors the flavors of a caprese salad in an unexpectedly melty way. Named after the island of Capri, the caprese salad hails from the Campania region of southern Italy. In the shadow of Mount Vesuvius, the area's volcanic soil is vibrantly fertile and rich in minerals, producing flavorful plum tomatoes that perfectly balance this salad's wonderfully creamy and juicy costar, fresh mozzarella. When broiled on a piece of bread, the caprese flavors marry and the bread slightly toasts, creating a rustic meal that comforts the soul.

SERVES 2 • PREP TIME: 10 minutes • **COOK TIME:** 5 minutes

1 cup diced tomatoes

1 cup diced fresh mozza-
rella cheese

1 tablespoon extra-virgin
olive oil

½ teaspoon salt

2 slices Basic Bread
(page 117)

1 tablespoon bal-
samic vinegar

4 fresh basil leaves, chopped

TIP: When fresh mozzarella isn't available, mix
2 tablespoons of cream
cheese into 1 cup of
shredded mozzarella
to mimic fresh mozza-
rella's creamy texture.
A grind of pepper and
an extra pinch of salt
will bring all the flavors
together. *Mangia!*

1 Preheat the oven to broil. Arrange a rack to the highest position (or closest to the broiler). Line a baking sheet with parchment paper.

2 In a small bowl, combine the tomatoes, mozzarella, olive oil, and salt. Marinate for about 10 minutes to let the flavors combine.

3 Drain and reserve any excess juice that accumulates in the bottom of the bowl. (Don't waste it. Use it in salad dressings or to flavor vegetable soup.)

4 Arrange the bread slices cut-side up on the baking sheet. Place half of the tomato mixture on each slice of bread. Broil until the mozzarella is melted, about 2 minutes.

5 Remove from the oven and top each open-faced sandwich with a drizzle of balsamic vinegar and a sprinkle of chopped basil.

PER SERVING (1 OPEN-FACED SANDWICH): Calories: 410;
Total fat: 34g; Protein: 17g; Total carbs: 9g; Fiber: 3g;
Net carbs: 6g

MACROS: Fat: 75%; Protein: 16%; Carbs: 9%

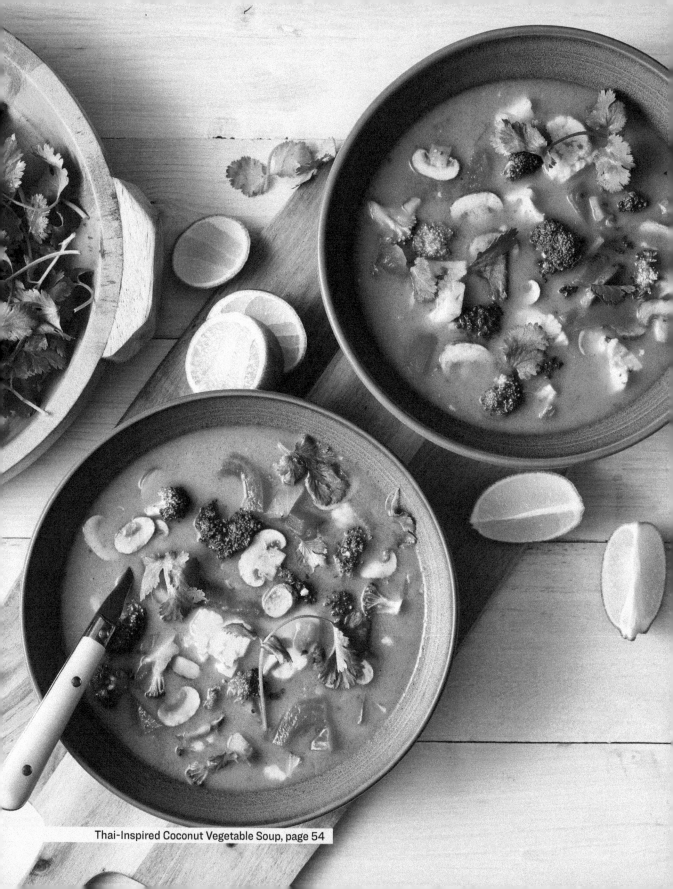

Thai-Inspired Coconut Vegetable Soup, page 54

CHAPTER 4

Soups, Stews, and Chilis

Asparagus and White Cheddar Soup   EF   5   GF   NF   Q   SF 52

Coconut Leek Soup   GF   OP   V 53

Thai-Inspired Coconut Vegetable Soup   GF   OP   Q   SF   V 54

Cream of Mushroom Soup   EF   GF   NF   Q   SF 55

Cheesy Curried Cauliflower Chowder   EF   GF   NF   SF 56

Sesame Bok Choy Ramen   NF   OP   Q   V 58

Green Chile Stew   GF   NF   Q   SF   V 59

Chipotle Chili   GF   NF   OP   SF   V 60

Ratatouille   GF   NF   SF   V 61

Ribollita   GF   SF 62

Asparagus and White Cheddar Soup

Cream of asparagus soup is a longtime favorite. When I am feeling particularly decadent, the addition of white cheddar takes this easy soup from a 10 to 11.

SERVES 4 • PREP TIME: 5 minutes • COOK TIME: 25 minutes

2 tablespoons butter

2 cups diced fresh
   asparagus

½ cup Vegetable
   Broth (page 108) or
   store-bought vegeta-
   ble broth

1 cup heavy whipping cream

1 cup shredded
   white cheddar

1 In a large pot over medium heat, melt the butter. Add the asparagus and sauté until tender, stirring occasionally, about 5 minutes.

2 Add the broth and the cream. Increase the heat to high and bring to a boil. Reduce the heat to medium-low and simmer for 10 to 15 minutes, until slightly thickened.

3 Carefully transfer half the soup to a blender and puree until smooth.

4 Return the blended soup to the pot. Add the cheddar and simmer, uncovered, for 5 minutes or until the cheese is melted.

TIP: Use caution when adding hot liquids to a blender. Fill the blender no more than halfway, remove the center cap from the blender lid, place a dishtowel over the blender lid, and start on a slow speed.

PER SERVING (1 CUP): Calories: 381; Total fat: 37g; Protein: 10g; Total carbs: 5g; Fiber: 1g; Net carbs: 4g

MACROS: Fat: 87%; Protein: 10%; Carbs: 3%

Coconut Leek Soup

To stay current with low-carb trends, I routinely scour the Internet to learn what my peers are promoting and how we can collaborate to influence healthy vegetarian keto behaviors. This recipe is a savory contribution from the bloggers behind Castle in the Mountains, *a husband-and-wife team who specialize in easy keto recipes for the low-carb lifestyle. Coconut leek soup is an all-season, well-spiced soup with fresh flavors and creamy tofu. Enjoy it as a nutritious, complete meal with a green salad and low-carb bread or as a starter for a hearty meal.*

SERVES 8 • PREP TIME: 15 minutes **• COOK TIME:** 35 minutes

2 tablespoons olive oil

3 cups thinly sliced leeks

¾ cup thinly sliced carrot

1 clove garlic, minced

4 cups Vegetable Broth (page 108) or store-bought vegetable broth

12 ounces firm tofu, cubed

1 cup thinly sliced celery

1 teaspoon curry powder

1 teaspoon grated fresh ginger or ½ teaspoon ground ginger

½ teaspoon ground turmeric

⅛ teaspoon freshly ground black pepper

Pinch red pepper flakes

1 (13-ounce) can unsweetened full-fat coconut milk

Fresh basil leaves, fresh cilantro, sliced bell peppers, and lime wedges, for garnish (optional)

1 In a large pot over medium heat, heat the oil. Add the leeks, carrot, and garlic and sauté until fragrant and beginning to soften, about 5 minutes.

2 Add the broth, tofu, celery, curry powder, ginger, turmeric, black pepper, and red pepper flakes to the pot. Stir to combine. Cover and simmer for about 30 minutes or until the vegetables are tender. Taste for seasoning.

3 Add the coconut milk and heat until just hot. Do not allow to boil once the coconut milk has been added.

4 Serve as is or with your desired garnishes.

TIP: Replace the tofu with an equal amount of sliced mushrooms, if you prefer.

PER SERVING (1 CUP): Calories: 165; Total fat: 13g; Protein: 5g; Total carbs: 6g; Fiber: 1g; Net carbs: 5g

MACROS: Fat: 71%; Protein: 12%; Carbs: 17%

Thai-Inspired Coconut Vegetable Soup

If you've ever been to a Thai restaurant, this take on tom yum soup may be familiar. This recipe is the vegan keto version of the classic Thai dish. For a lighter version of this soup, omit the coconut cream. A good substitute is half an avocado to ensure you're getting plenty of healthy fat.

SERVES 4 • PREP TIME: 10 minutes **• COOK TIME:** 20 minutes

8 cups Vegetable Broth (page 108) or store-bought vegetable broth

1 teaspoon ground ginger

2 cloves garlic, diced

1 lime, zested and cut into wedges

1 cup full-fat coconut cream

1 cup sliced mushrooms

1 cup coarsely chopped broccoli florets

1 cup coarsely chopped cauliflower florets

1 tomato, coarsely chopped

½ medium yellow onion, coarsely chopped

1 cup chopped fresh cilantro, optional, for garnish

1 In a large stockpot over medium heat, combine the broth, ginger, garlic, and lime zest. Bring to a simmer.

2 Add the coconut cream, followed by the mushrooms, broccoli, cauliflower, tomato, and onion. Simmer until the vegetables are tender, about 15 minutes.

3 Remove the pot from the heat and serve the soup garnished with the cilantro (if using) and lime wedges.

PER SERVING (¼ RECIPE): Calories: 97; Total fat: 7g; Protein: 1g; Total carbs: 9g; Fiber: 3g; Net carbs: 6g

MACROS: Fat: 65%; Protein: 4%; Carbs: 31%

Cream of Mushroom Soup

EF

GF

NF

Q

SF

Cream of mushroom soup isn't just for green bean casserole. In fact, all creamed vegetable soups follow roughly the same makeup: an aromatic (onion or leek), a prominent vegetable (broccoli or asparagus), and a creamy element (dairy or nondairy). Puree it all together and you have a warming soup that will bring everyone to the table.

SERVES 2 • PREP TIME: 10 minutes • **COOK TIME:** 20 minutes

4 tablespoons butter

2 cups sliced mushrooms

1 teaspoon freshly ground black pepper

½ teaspoon salt

¼ cup minced shallot (about 1 large shallot)

1 teaspoon minced garlic

4 cups Vegetable Broth (page 108) or store-bought vegetable broth

½ cup heavy cream

1 teaspoon dried thyme

1 In a medium pot over medium heat, melt the butter. Add the mushrooms and cook for 5 minutes, until softened. Season with the pepper and salt. Remove ¼ cup of mushrooms and reserve in a small bowl.

2 To the pot, add the shallot and garlic and cook for 2 to 3 minutes, until tender. Add the broth, cream, and thyme. Increase the heat to high and bring to a boil.

3 Reduce the heat to medium-low and simmer for 10 minutes, until slightly thickened.

4 Carefully transfer the soup to a blender and puree until smooth. Ladle into two bowls and garnish with the reserved mushrooms.

PER SERVING (½ RECIPE): Calories: 452; Total fat: 45g; Protein: 5g; Total carbs: 11g; Fiber: 2g; Net carbs: 9g

MACROS: Fat: 90%; Protein: 4%; Carbs: 6%

Cheesy Curried Cauliflower Chowder

I am very inspired by Indian food and flavors, particularly because vegetarianism is deeply embedded in Indian culture. Although most of the curried cauliflower dishes I've enjoyed in the past feature coconut milk, this unique preparation is dairy-forward with heavy cream and mozzarella, creating a rich, velvety chowder.

SERVES 4 • PREP TIME: 10 minutes • **COOK TIME:** 55 minutes

1 small head cauliflower, cored and cut into florets

1 tablespoon olive oil

1 tablespoon curry powder

½ teaspoon salt

½ teaspoon freshly ground black pepper

3 tablespoons butter

½ cup chopped shallots (about 2 large shallots)

1 teaspoon minced garlic

½ cup chopped carrots

½ cup chopped celery

3 cups Vegetable Broth (page 108) or store-bought vegetable broth

1 bay leaf

½ teaspoon ground turmeric

1 cup heavy cream

¾ cup shredded mozzarella cheese, divided

1 Preheat the oven to 400°F. Line a baking sheet with parchment paper.

2 On the baking sheet, toss the cauliflower in the olive oil and season with the curry powder, salt, and pepper.

3 Spread the cauliflower into a single layer and roast until tender, about 30 minutes. Set aside to cool.

4 In a large pot over medium heat, melt the butter. Add the shallots and garlic and cook for 2 minutes, until softened.

5 Add the carrots and celery and cook for 5 minutes, stirring occasionally, until softened. Add the roasted curried cauliflower, broth, bay leaf, and turmeric.

6 Bring to a boil, then reduce the heat to low and simmer for 10 minutes, until the vegetables are tender.

7　Remove the bay leaf. Using a ladle, carefully transfer about 1 cup of soup (½ cup of broth and ½ cup of vegetables) to a blender. Blend until completely smooth, then return to the pot. Simmer for another 10 minutes until the flavors have mingled.

8　Add the cream and ½ cup of mozzarella. Continue simmering, stirring frequently, for 2 to 3 minutes until the mozzarella has melted.

9　Ladle the chowder into bowls and garnish each with 1 tablespoon of the remaining shredded mozzarella.

TIP: The yellow color of curry powder comes from ground turmeric. Turmeric is high in anti-inflammatory properties, making it especially comforting after a tough workout.

PER SERVING (¼ RECIPE): Calories: 409; Total fat: 37g; Protein: 8g; Total carbs: 14g; Fiber: 4g; Net carbs: 10g

MACROS: Fat: 81%; Protein: 8%; Carbs: 11%

Sesame Bok Choy Ramen

My simple formula for Asian-inspired soup is broth plus soy sauce plus sesame oil. Add virtually any protein, vegetable, and/or noodle, and you have a homemade soup on the table faster than you could pick up takeout. When I am in a spicy mood, I drizzle sriracha over the top for an extra punch.

SERVES 2 • PREP TIME: 5 minutes **• COOK TIME:** 15 minutes

1 teaspoon olive oil

1 head baby bok choy, sliced

¼ cup thinly sliced carrots

1 teaspoon minced garlic

1 teaspoon grated
    fresh ginger

4 cups Vegetable
    Broth (page 108)
    or store-bought
    vegetable broth

2 tablespoons soy sauce

2 teaspoons sesame oil

1 (7-ounce) package shira-
    taki noodles

1 tablespoon thinly sliced
    scallions, white and
    green parts

1 In a medium pot over medium-high heat, heat the olive oil until shimmering. Add the bok choy and carrots and cook for 5 minutes, stirring frequently, until softened.

2 Reduce the heat to medium and add the garlic and ginger. Cook for 30 seconds until fragrant.

3 Add the broth, soy sauce, and sesame oil. Scrape the bottom of the pot to release any vegetables that may be stuck.

4 Increase the heat to high and bring to a boil, then reduce the heat to medium-low and simmer for 5 minutes, until the flavors marry.

5 Prepare the shirataki noodles according to the package instructions. Add the noodles to the broth.

6 Serve each bowl with a sprinkle of scallions.

TIP: Although shirataki noodles are packed in water, they might smell a bit strange when you open the package. This is because they are made with konjac root, which naturally has a slightly fishy smell. To remove the smell, simply rinse the noodles very well under cold running water before you prepare them.

PER SERVING (½ RECIPE): Calories: 115; Total fat: 8g; Protein: 4g; Total carbs: 10g; Fiber: 2g; Net carbs: 8g

MACROS: Fat: 63%; Protein: 14%; Carbs: 23%

Green Chile Stew

There's more than one way to thicken a soup or stew. My trick is to puree water and nuts or seeds to add high-fat, low-carb body and complexity. In this case, pumpkin seeds are a natural choice because they are traditionally paired with green chiles to prepare a Pueblan classic called pipián verde.

GF
NF
Q
SF
V

SERVES 2 • PREP TIME: 5 minutes • **COOK TIME:** 25 minutes

1 tablespoon olive oil

¼ cup diced shallot (about 1 large shallot)

¼ teaspoon salt, plus more for seasoning

1 teaspoon sweet paprika

1 teaspoon ground cumin

½ teaspoon dried oregano

2 tablespoons minced jalapeño pepper

2 cups Vegetable Broth (page 108) or store-bought vegetable broth

2 (4-ounce) cans diced green chiles

4 tablespoons shelled pumpkin seeds

½ cup water

2 tablespoons freshly squeezed lime juice

Freshly ground black pepper

2 tablespoons chopped fresh cilantro

1 avocado, peeled, pitted, and diced

1 In a medium pot over medium heat, heat the olive oil until shimmering. Add the shallot and salt and sauté for 5 minutes, until softened.

2 Stir in the paprika, cumin, oregano, and jalapeño and cook for an additional 2 minutes. Add the broth and diced green chiles. Bring to a boil, then reduce to a simmer.

3 In a blender, combine the pumpkin seeds and ½ cup of water. Puree until smooth. Add the pureed pumpkin seeds to the simmering stew and continue to cook, stirring occasionally, for 10 to 15 minutes, until thickened.

4 Remove the stew from the heat, stir in the lime juice, and season to taste with salt and pepper.

5 Garnish with the cilantro and avocado and serve.

TIP: If your lifestyle permits dairy products, consider a drizzle of Mexican crema. Less acidic than sour cream, crema is thinner and is less likely to curdle over warm dishes.

PER SERVING (½ RECIPE): Calories: 314; Total fat: 25g; Protein: 11g; Total carbs: 20g; Fiber: 7g; Net carbs: 13g

MACROS: Fat: 72%; Protein: 14%; Carbs: 14%

GF
NF
OP
SF
V

Chipotle Chili

"Chili" and "vegetarian" aren't typically used in the same sentence—but that doesn't mean they can't be besties. The undisputed star of this dish is the chipotle in adobo, a spicy smoked chile bathed in a deep red, tangy sauce. There are generally a few chipotle peppers per 7-ounce can. To preserve the remaining chipotles, place them in a resealable freezer-safe container and freeze for up to six months.

SERVES 2 • PREP TIME: 5 minutes • **COOK TIME:** 35 minutes

1 tablespoon olive oil

1 celery stalk, diced

1 tablespoon chili powder

1 tablespoon ground cumin

1 teaspoon dried oregano

½ teaspoon minced garlic

1 cup diced cauliflower

½ cup diced bell pepper, any color

½ cup diced zucchini

1 cup diced tomatoes (fresh or canned)

1 cup water

1 tablespoon minced chipotle in adobo

1 tablespoon tomato paste

½ teaspoon salt

½ teaspoon freshly ground black pepper

1 avocado, peeled, pitted, and diced

¼ cup sliced radishes

2 tablespoons chopped fresh cilantro

1 In a medium pot over medium heat, heat the olive oil until shimmering. Add the celery and cook for 3 minutes, until softened. Add the chili powder, cumin, oregano, and garlic. Cook and stir for 2 more minutes.

2 Add the cauliflower, bell pepper, and zucchini and cook for 10 minutes, stirring occasionally, until softened.

3 Add the tomatoes, water, chipotle, tomato paste, salt, and pepper. Reduce the heat to medium-low and simmer for 20 minutes, until the vegetables are tender.

4 Ladle the chili into bowls and serve each with half the avocado, 2 tablespoons sliced radishes, and 1 tablespoon cilantro.

TIP: If you prefer a chili with a stew-like consistency, mash some of the vegetables or puree 1 to 2 cups of the chili in a blender to even out the texture.

PER SERVING (½ RECIPE): Calories: 279; Total fat: 19g; Protein: 7g; Total carbs: 26g; Fiber: 12g; Net carbs: 14g

MACROS: Fat: 61%; Protein: 10%; Carbs: 29%

Ratatouille

GF

NF

SF

V

We have the south of France to thank for ratatouille, which is often served in late summer when zucchini and eggplant are at their peak. As the daughter of a Frenchman, I honor the tradition of cooking each vegetable separately, then marrying them together. However, feel free to cut the cooking time by sautéing all the vegetables together.

SERVES 4 • PREP TIME: 10 minutes **• COOK TIME:** 45 minutes

3 tablespoons olive oil, divided

2 cups diced and peeled eggplant

1 teaspoon salt, divided

1 teaspoon freshly ground black pepper, divided

2 cups diced zucchini

½ cup diced shallots (about 2 large shallots)

1 teaspoon minced garlic

1 thyme sprig

1 bay leaf

20 grape tomatoes, quartered

2 tablespoons torn fresh basil

TIP: If liquid accumulates in the bottom of the pot, increase the heat until it evaporates. Ratatouille is not meant to be soupy and should be stirred frequently.

1 In a large pot over medium-high heat, heat 1 tablespoon olive oil until shimmering. Add the eggplant, ½ teaspoon salt, and ½ teaspoon pepper. Cook for 5 minutes, stirring occasionally, until softened. Transfer to a large bowl.

2 To the pot, add 1 tablespoon olive oil and the zucchini. Season with the remaining salt and pepper and cook for 3 minutes, stirring occasionally, until softened. Transfer to the eggplant bowl.

3 Reduce the heat to medium. Add the remaining 1 tablespoon olive oil and the shallots. Cook for 5 minutes, stirring occasionally, until fragrant. Add the garlic, thyme, and bay leaf and cook for 1 minute, stirring constantly. Add the tomatoes and return the eggplant and zucchini to the pot. Stir gently to combine.

4 Reduce the heat to medium-low and simmer for 30 minutes, stirring occasionally, until the vegetables are tender. Remove the bay leaf and thyme sprig. Stir in the basil just before serving.

PER SERVING (¼ RECIPE): Calories: 137; Total fat: 11g; Protein: 2g; Total carbs: 10g; Fiber: 3g; Net carbs: 7g

MACROS: Fat: 72%; Protein: 6%; Carbs: 22%

Ribollita

Authentic ribollita is a Tuscan soup that features vegetables, white can-nellini beans, and crusty bread. A symbol of cucina povera, *or Italian peasant food, ribollita means "twice boiled" and is traditionally made with leftover minestrone. My version of ribollita skips the cannellini beans but preserves the bread in a richly seasoned vegetable stew that always brings me back to the rolling hills of Tuscany.*

SERVES 4 • PREP TIME: 10 minutes • **COOK TIME:** 45 minutes

4 tablespoons extra-virgin olive oil, divided

2 cups shredded laci-nato kale

1 cup quartered grape tomatoes

½ cup diced shallots (about 2 large shallots)

½ cup diced carrot

1 teaspoon minced garlic plus 1 whole clove, peeled

½ teaspoon salt

½ teaspoon freshly ground black pepper

1 teaspoon tomato paste

3 cups Vegetable Broth (page 108) or store-bought vegetable broth

1 teaspoon dried oregano

1 bay leaf

1 small vegetarian Par-mesan cheese rind plus 4 teaspoons grated vege-tarian Parmesan

4 slices Basic Bread (page 117)

1   In a large pot over medium heat, heat 2 tablespoons of oil until shimmering. Add the kale, tomatoes, shallots, carrot, minced garlic, salt, and pepper. Cook for 7 to 10 minutes, until the vegetables are tender.

2   Add the tomato paste and stir for about 30 seconds. Add the broth and scrape the bottom of the pot to release anything that is sticking. Add the oregano, bay leaf, and Parmesan rind. Increase the heat to high and bring to a boil.

3   Reduce the heat to low and simmer for 30 minutes, until the vegetables are very soft. (Use this time to prepare the Basic Bread.) Remove the bay leaf and Parmesan rind.

4   Toast the Basic Bread slices until golden brown. Lightly brush them with olive oil (about 1 tablespoon total) and gently rub each piece with the whole garlic clove.

5 Place the toasts in four serving bowls and ladle the soup over the toasts. Drizzle each bowl with the remaining olive oil and sprinkle with grated Parmesan.

TIP: Although lacinato kale is traditional for ribollita, you can substitute other varieties of kale or even cabbage.

PER SERVING (1 BOWL): Calories: 350; Total fat: 30g; Protein: 10g; Total carbs: 18g; Fiber: 5g; Net carbs: 13g

MACROS: Fat: 77%; Protein: 11%; Carbs: 12%

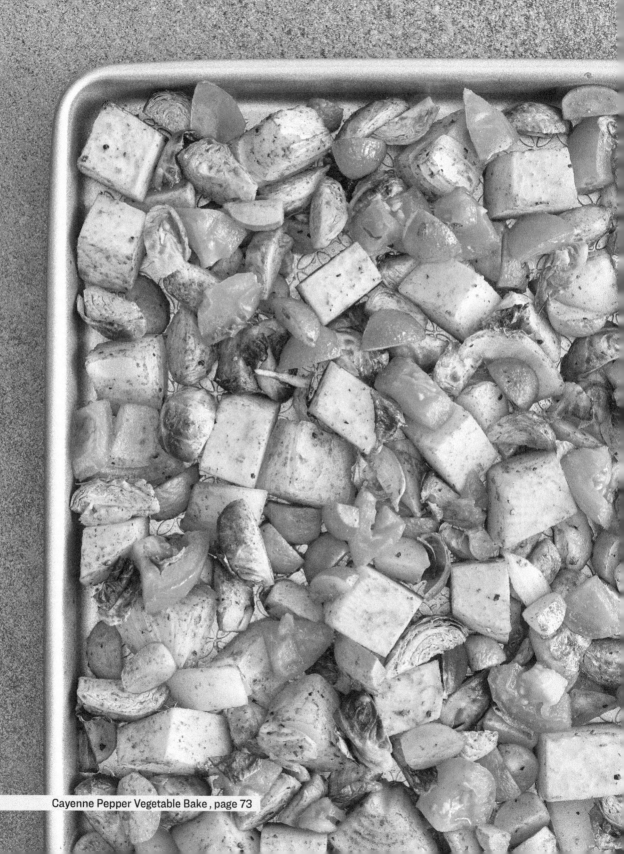

Cayenne Pepper Vegetable Bake , page 73

CHAPTER 5

Mains

Shirataki Florentine EF GF NF Q SF 66

Eggplant Marinara GF SF 67

Wild Mushroom Tofu Ragù EF GF NF OP 68

Portabella Mushroom Margherita Pizza EF 5 GF NF Q SF 69

Crustless Spanakopita GF SF 70

Green Bean and Mushroom Casserole GF OP SF V 72

Cayenne Pepper Vegetable Bake GF NF OP SF V 73

Spaghetti Squash Egg Bake GF NF SF 74

Buffalo "Mac-and-Cheese" Bake EF SF 76

Casserole Relleno 5 GF NF SF 77

Garlic Fried Cauliflower Rice GF NF Q V 78

Egg Foo Young DF GF NF SF 79

Thai-Inspired Peanut Roasted Cauliflower GF Q SF V 80

Egg Cauliflower Tikka Masala GF NF OP SF 81

Shirataki Florentine

Shirataki is a delicate, plant-based super noodle that literally nets out to zero carbs—the perfect keto food. Full disclosure: The first time I tried shirataki noodles, I could not get past their texture. But I soon learned that was because I had not thoroughly rinsed them as the package suggests. I also neglected to place them in a pan (no oil or butter) over medium heat until they were thoroughly dry. These steps are critical to ensuring the texture of the noodles is pasta-like—a must for this Italian preparation.

SERVES 2 • PREP TIME: 5 minutes • **COOK TIME:** 20 minutes

2 tablespoons unsalted butter

2 teaspoons minced garlic

1 shallot, minced

⅓ cup Vegetable Broth (page 108) or store-bought vegetable broth

4 cups fresh spinach

½ cup heavy cream

2 tablespoons grated vegetarian Parmesan

½ teaspoon salt

½ teaspoon freshly ground pepper

1 (7-ounce) package shirataki noodles

1 In a large skillet over medium heat, melt the butter. Add the garlic and shallot and sauté for 2 minutes, stirring frequently, until softened.

2 Add the broth and simmer for 3 minutes. Then add the spinach and wilt for about 1 minute.

3 Reduce the heat to medium-low and add the cream and Parmesan. Simmer for 3 to 5 minutes until thickened, then add the salt and pepper.

4 Prepare the shirataki noodles according to the package instructions. Reduce the heat to low and add the noodles to the pan. Simmer for 5 minutes to warm through, then serve.

TIP: Parmesan tastes best when it's freshly grated; however, there are numerous high-quality brands of pre-grated Parmesan available in the refrigerated section of the grocery store, near the fresh pasta.

PER SERVING (½ RECIPE): Calories: 374; Total fat: 35g; Protein: 6g; Total carbs: 12g; Fiber: 4g; Net carbs: 8g

MACROS: Fat: 84%; Protein: 6%; Carbs: 10%

Eggplant Marinara

Eggplant is a real workhorse ingredient. It takes on a "meaty" texture when cooked, and it's also surprisingly versatile. This recipe uses keto-friendly almond flour in place of bread crumbs to coat the cutlets, which are then topped with zesty marinara sauce.

SERVES 4 • PREP TIME: 20 minutes • **COOK TIME:** 1 hour

½ cup almond flour

1 teaspoon salt

1 teaspoon minced garlic

1 teaspoon onion powder

2 large eggs

6 tablespoons olive oil

1 eggplant, cut into ⅓-inch-thick rounds

1 cup sliced mushrooms

1 (10-ounce) bag spinach

1 (8-ounce) block cream cheese, cubed

1 (24-ounce) jar low-carb, no-sugar-added marinara sauce (such as Rao's Homemade)

1 Preheat the oven to 350°F.

2 In a medium bowl, mix together the almond flour, salt, garlic, and onion powder.

3 In another bowl, beat the eggs for dipping.

4 In a large skillet over medium-high heat, heat the oil until shimmering.

5 One at a time, dip the eggplant slices, first in the eggs and then in the flour mixture, turning to coat. Transfer to the skillet and cook for 2 to 3 minutes per side, until golden brown.

6 Once the eggplant slices are browned, arrange them in a single layer in a large baking dish. When the bottom of the baking dish is covered, add layers of mushrooms, spinach, and cream cheese. Top with a second layer of browned eggplant, mushrooms, spinach, and cream cheese. Continue making layers until you run out of ingredients.

7 Pour the marinara sauce over the top of the layers.

8 Bake for 40 minutes or until the sauce is bubbling.

PER SERVING (¼ RECIPE): Calories: 668; Total fat: 60g; Protein: 15g; Total carbs: 23g; Fiber: 8g; Net carbs: 15g

MACROS: Fat: 81%; Protein: 9%; Carbs: 10%

Wild Mushroom Tofu Ragù

Mushrooms have an earthy taste that complements the heavy cream, garlic, and thyme in this stew. You may only think of herbs in terms of flavor, but these little plants are also superfoods. Thyme, for instance, is high in volatile oils and flavonoids as well as vitamin K and iron. Be generous with the thyme, and your body will thank you.

SERVES 4 • PREP TIME: 15 minutes • **COOK TIME:** 25 minutes

3 tablespoons olive oil

2 zucchini, diced

1 medium yellow onion, chopped

1 tablespoon minced garlic

1 pound assorted wild mushrooms, sliced

8 ounces extra-firm tofu, pressed

1 cup heavy (whipping) cream

½ cup Vegetable Broth (page 108) or store-bought vegetable broth

2 teaspoons chopped fresh thyme

Sea salt

Freshly ground black pepper

1 In a large skillet over medium-high heat, heat the oil until shimmering. Add the zucchini, onion, and garlic and sauté until tender, about 6 minutes.

2 Stir in the mushrooms and tofu and sauté until the liquid purges and the mushrooms caramelize, about 10 minutes.

3 Stir in the heavy cream, broth, and thyme and bring the ragù to a boil. Reduce the heat to low and simmer until the sauce thickens, about 6 minutes.

4 Season with salt and pepper and serve.

TIP: For a vegan-friendly option, swap the heavy cream for the same amount of coconut milk and add a scoop of vegan protein powder. This will change the calories to 395 per serving and the macros to Fat: 71%; Protein: 20%; Carbs: 9%.

PER SERVING (¼ RECIPE): Calories: 456; Total fat: 40g; Protein: 15g; Total carbs: 9g; Fiber: 3g; Net carbs: 6g

MACROS: Fat: 79%; Protein: 13%; Carbs: 8%

Portabella Mushroom Margherita Pizza

EF

5

GF

NF

Q

SF

Portabella mushrooms have a meaty texture that soaks up spices, herbs, and other flavorings like a sponge. It's no wonder they're a main course in many vegan and vegetarian restaurants. Mushrooms are a rare vegetable source of vitamin D and also contain high levels of potassium. The fats (cheese and olive oil) in this recipe help you absorb that all-important vitamin D.

SERVES 4 • PREP TIME: 15 minutes • **COOK TIME:** 10 minutes

¾ cup olive oil

2 teaspoons minced garlic

6 large portabella mushrooms, stems removed

1½ cups low-carb, no-sugar-added marinara sauce (such as Rao's Homemade)

3 cups shredded mozzarella cheese

3 tablespoons chopped fresh basil, for garnish

1 Preheat the oven to broil. Line a baking sheet with aluminum foil and set aside.

2 In a medium bowl, stir together the olive oil and garlic, then add the mushrooms. Rub the oil all over the mushrooms and place them gill-side down on the prepared baking sheet.

3 Broil the mushrooms until they are tender, turning once, about 4 minutes total.

4 Remove the baking sheet from the oven and evenly divide the marinara sauce among the mushroom caps, spreading it on the gill side. Then top with the mozzarella cheese.

5 Return the sheet to the oven and broil the mushrooms until the cheese is melted and bubbly, 1 to 2 minutes. Serve topped with basil.

TIP: If you're not vegetarian, pepperoni, Italian sausage, and prosciutto are delectable additions to these hearty pizzas. Meat will add protein and a few grams of fat to the dish.

PER SERVING (2 MUSHROOMS): Calories: 325; Total fat: 25g; Protein: 16g; Total carbs: 9g; Fiber: 3g; Net carbs: 6g

MACROS: Fat: 69%; Protein: 20%; Carbs: 11%

Crustless Spanakopita

Spanakopita is a savory Greek pie with a spinach and feta filling inside a flaky phyllo crust. Most versions found in the United States are heavy on the crust and light on the filling. This crustless version is heavy on the spinach and adds fresh ricotta and eggs for texture and protein. It's a delicious vegetarian meal on its own or you can serve it alongside a light soup for something heartier.

SERVES 6 • PREP TIME: 15 minutes • **COOK TIME:** 55 minutes

12 tablespoons olive oil, divided

1 small yellow onion, diced

1 (32-ounce) bag frozen chopped spinach, thawed, fully drained, and patted dry (about 4 cups)

4 cloves garlic, minced

½ teaspoon salt

½ teaspoon freshly ground black pepper

4 large eggs

1 cup whole-milk ricotta cheese

¾ cup crumbled traditional feta cheese

¼ cup pine nuts

1 Preheat the oven to 375°F.

2 In a large skillet over medium-high heat, heat 4 tablespoons olive oil until shimmering. Add the onion and sauté until softened, 6 to 8 minutes.

3 Add the spinach, garlic, salt, and pepper and sauté another 5 minutes. Remove from the heat and allow to cool slightly.

4 In a medium bowl, whisk together the eggs and ricotta. Add to the cooled spinach and stir to combine.

5 Pour 4 tablespoons olive oil into a 9-by-13-inch glass baking dish and swirl to coat the bottom and sides. Add the spinach-ricotta mixture and spread into an even layer.

6 Bake for 20 minutes or until the mixture begins to set. Remove from the oven and crumble the feta evenly across the top of the spinach. Add the pine nuts and drizzle with the remaining 4 tablespoons olive oil.

7 Return to the oven and bake for an additional 15 to 20 minutes or until the spinach is fully set and the top is starting to turn golden brown. Allow to cool slightly before cutting to serve.

TIP: Traditional Greek feta is made from sheep's milk and typically found in block form, but much of the commercial feta in the United States is made from cow's milk and sold crumbled. The flavor of the traditional version is far superior and worth seeking out. Substitute goat cheese if you prefer a less salty flavor.

PER SERVING: Calories: 484, Total fat: 43g, Protein: 18g; Total carbs: 10g, Fiber: 5g; Net carbs: 5g

MACROS: Fat: 79%; Protein: 13%; Carbs: 8%

Green Bean and Mushroom Casserole

The green bean casserole is a classic that you might only associate with Thanksgiving, but you'll want this version to make regular appearances on your table all year round. The casserole has fresh green beans and mushrooms, a rich, creamy sauce, and a crunchy topping of slivered almonds. What more could you want?

SERVES 6 • PREP TIME: 15 minutes • **COOK TIME:** 1 hour

2 tablespoons olive oil, divided

1 pound fresh green beans, trimmed and cut into 2- to 3-inch lengths

12 ounces mushrooms, sliced

1 yellow onion, diced

1 shallot, diced

1 (13-ounce) can unsweetened full-fat coconut milk

½ cup Vegetable Broth (page 108) or store-bought vegetable broth

3 tablespoons minced garlic

1 teaspoon salt

1 teaspoon freshly ground black pepper

½ cup slivered almonds

1 Preheat the oven to 350°F. Grease a 9-by-13-inch baking dish with 1 tablespoon oil.

2 In the prepared baking dish, toss the green beans, mushrooms, onion, and shallot together with the remaining 1 tablespoon oil.

3 Pour the coconut milk and broth over the vegetables, and add the garlic, salt, and pepper. Stir gently to mix. Sprinkle the slivered almonds over the top.

4 Bake for 1 hour or until the vegetables are tender.

PER SERVING (⅙ RECIPE): Calories: 253; Total fat: 20g; Protein: 6g; Total carbs: 16g; Fiber: 5g; Net carbs: 9g

MACROS: Fat: 71%; Protein: 9%; Carbs: 20%

Cayenne Pepper Vegetable Bake

GF
NF
OP
SF
V

Make a big pan of baked vegetables at the beginning of the week and eat them all week long as a side dish, topped with fried eggs for a quick breakfast-for-dinner, or on their own as a light meal. Brussels sprouts work well for this kind of dish because they're sturdy enough to hold up during the long bake without turning mushy. Their leafy edges tend to brown and crisp up, giving the dish an appetizing texture. Adjust the amount of cayenne in this vegetarian bake to your taste—if you really love heat, you could go up to ¼ cup.

SERVES 12 • PREP TIME: 20 minutes • **COOK TIME:** 1 hour

1 bunch Brussels sprouts (about 20), stemmed and diced

1 bunch radishes (about 12), diced

2 turnips, peeled and diced

1 tomato, diced

1 yellow onion, diced

6 tablespoons olive oil

2 tablespoons cayenne pepper

2 teaspoons salt

1 teaspoon freshly ground black pepper

1 Preheat the oven to 400°F.

2 On a large rimmed baking sheet, combine the Brussels sprouts, radishes, turnips, tomato, and onion. Add the olive oil and toss to coat well. Season with the cayenne, salt, and pepper.

3 Bake for 1 hour or until the vegetables are browned and crisp. Store, covered, in the refrigerator for up to 1 week.

TIP: Make this dish your own by substituting different vegetables. Broccoli, cauliflower, or asparagus could all take the place of the Brussels sprouts—or just add them to the mix. You may need to adjust the cooking time a bit when using more delicate vegetables.

PER SERVING (¹⁄₁₂ RECIPE): Calories: 89; Total fat: 7g; Protein: 2g; Total carbs: 6g; Fiber: 2g; Net carbs: 4g

MACROS: Fat: 71%; Protein: 9%; Carbs: 20%

Spaghetti Squash Egg Bake

If you've never had spaghetti squash before, you're in for a treat. Once cooked, it pulls apart into strands that mimic pasta. Spaghetti squash is also a fabulous source of beta-carotene, potassium, calcium, and vitamins A, B, and C. The squash pairs beautifully with the egg-and-cream base baked into this casserole.

SERVES 4 • PREP TIME: 15 minutes • **COOK TIME:** 1 hour 10 minutes

2 tablespoons olive oil, plus more for greasing

1 spaghetti squash, halved lengthwise and seeded

1 cup water

½ yellow onion, chopped

1 teaspoon minced garlic

6 large eggs

2 ounces cream cheese

1 tablespoon chopped fresh basil

Sea salt

Freshly ground black pepper

1 cup grated vegetarian Parmesan cheese

1 Preheat the oven to 375°F. Lightly grease a 9-by-13-inch casserole dish with olive oil.

2 Place the squash cut-side down in a baking dish that fits inside your microwave and add 1 cup of water. Microwave on high until a knife inserts easily into the flesh, 15 to 20 minutes.

3 Let the squash cool for 10 minutes and then shred the flesh with a fork into a large bowl.

4 While the squash is cooling, heat the remaining 2 tablespoons oil in a medium skillet over medium-high heat until shimmering. Add the onion and garlic and sauté until softened, about 3 minutes.

5 Add the onion to the bowl with the squash, followed by the eggs, cream cheese, and basil and mix until well combined. Season the mixture with salt and pepper.

6 Spoon the mixture into the prepared casserole dish and top evenly with the Parmesan cheese.

7 Cover the casserole loosely with aluminum foil and bake for 25 minutes, then remove the foil and bake until the eggs are cooked through and the top is golden, about 15 minutes more.

8 Let the casserole cool for 10 minutes before serving.

PER SERVING (¼ RECIPE): Calories: 363; Total fat: 27g; Protein: 19g; Total carbs: 11g; Fiber: 2g; Net carbs: 9g

MACROS: Fat: 67%; Protein: 20%; Carbs: 13%

Buffalo "Mac-and-Cheese" Bake

How's this for a twist on a classic? This mac-and-cheese bake has no mac, no shredded cheese, and an extra-spicy kick. Cauliflower takes on the noodle role, and cream cheese joins forces with nutritional yeast and coconut milk to do the rest of the work. Each bite is better than the last, especially with a tangy, creamy Buffalo-style sauce that will make you forget all about tradition.

SERVES 8 • PREP TIME: 20 minutes **• COOK TIME:** 1 hour

2 tablespoons olive oil, plus more for greasing

2 (8-ounce) blocks cream cheese

2 pounds grated cauliflower

1 yellow onion, diced

¾ cup sugar-free hot wing sauce (such as Frank's RedHot)

½ cup canned unsweetened full-fat coconut milk

2 tablespoons minced garlic

2 tablespoons nutritional yeast

1 teaspoon salt

1 teaspoon freshly ground black pepper

3 tablespoons chopped fresh chives

1 Preheat the oven to 400°F. Grease a 9-by-13-inch baking dish with oil.

2 In a large microwave-safe bowl, microwave the cream cheese on high for 1 minute until melted.

3 Into the bowl with the cream cheese, stir the cauliflower, onion, hot sauce, coconut milk, garlic, nutritional yeast, salt, and pepper. Mix well.

4 Transfer the mixture to the prepared baking dish. Drizzle the olive oil over the top.

5 Bake for 1 hour or until bubbly. Serve hot, topped with the chives.

PER SERVING (⅛ RECIPE): Calories: 311; Total fat: 26g; Protein: 8g; Total carbs: 13g; Fiber: 4g; Net carbs: 9g

MACROS: Fat: 75%; Protein: 10%; Carbs: 15%

Casserole Relleno

Chile relleno is one of my favorite dishes to order in a Mexican restaurant; however, it's generally deep-fried in a batter that isn't keto-friendly. This easy at-home version features canned green chiles, but if you have the time, save your canned chiles for Green Chile Stew (page 59) and roast a few poblano peppers at 400°F for 30 to 40 minutes for a smokier flavor.

SERVES 4 • PREP TIME: 10 minutes • **COOK TIME:** 40 minutes

Nonstick cooking spray

12 ounces canned whole green chiles, split open to lay flat

1 cup shredded cheddar cheese, divided

6 tablespoons crumbled cotija cheese, divided

2 eggs, beaten

½ teaspoon salt

¼ teaspoon freshly ground black pepper

1 Preheat the oven to 425°F. Coat the bottom of an 8-inch square baking dish with cooking spray.

2 Place a layer of chiles on the bottom of the dish. Cover the chiles with ½ cup of cheddar and 3 tablespoons of cotija.

3 Lay the remaining chiles over the cheese. Top with the remaining cheddar and cojita.

4 In a small bowl, combine the eggs, salt, and pepper and pour the egg mixture over the chiles and cheese.

5 Cover the baking dish with aluminum foil and bake for 40 minutes, until the cheese is bubbly. Cool for 10 minutes before serving.

TIP: If you can't find cotija cheese, feta cheese is a terrific substitute and offers a similar dry, crumbly texture and salty bite.

PER SERVING (¼ RECIPE): Calories: 214; Total fat: 15g; Protein: 12g; Total carbs: 7g; Fiber: 0g; Net carbs: 7g

MACROS: Fat: 63%; Protein: 22%; Carbs: 15%

Garlic Fried Cauliflower Rice

This "rice" dish provides everything you love about takeout without pushing you out of ketosis. It's also a great dish for entertaining. Make this in advance and store covered in your refrigerator, then pop in the oven at 350°F for 20 minutes to bring it up to temperature before serving.

SERVES 4 · PREP TIME: 10 minutes · **COOK TIME:** 20 minutes

1 (14-ounce) block sprouted tofu

4 tablespoons nutritional yeast

2 tablespoons tahini

1 teaspoon ground turmeric

1 teaspoon salt

1 tablespoon sesame oil

1 shallot, chopped

2 cloves garlic, minced

1 tablespoon ground ginger

1 cup chopped carrots

1 cup peas

6 cups grated cauliflower

½ cup chopped scallions (white and green parts), plus more for garnish

¼ cup tamari, plus more for drizzling

1 Drain the tofu, pressing it with a paper towel to absorb as much water as possible.

2 Into a medium mixing bowl, crumble the tofu. Add the nutritional yeast, tahini, turmeric, and salt and mix until it forms an egg-like texture.

3 In a large skillet over medium heat, heat the sesame oil until shimmering. Add the shallot, garlic, and ginger and cook, stirring regularly to prevent burning, until fragrant, about 3 minutes.

4 Add the carrots and peas and cook until the carrots become slightly tender, about 5 minutes. Add the tofu "eggs" to the skillet and toss. Allow the tofu to toast up slightly on each side.

5 Add the cauliflower, scallions, and tamari and stir thoroughly to mix all the flavors. Cook for 5 minutes to allow the flavors to meld and any excess liquid to cook off.

6 Remove from the heat, drizzle with tamari, and garnish with more chopped scallions.

PER SERVING (¼ RECIPE): Calories: 288; **Total fat:** 13g; **Protein:** 23g; **Total carbs:** 26g; **Fiber:** 9g; **Net carbs:** 17g

MACROS: Fat: 41%; **Protein:** 32%; **Carbs:** 27%

Egg Foo Young

This version of egg foo young is a ketogenic powerhouse. Cooked to a toasty golden brown, these egg patties are traditionally served with a high-carb brown gravy. My fresh spin preserves the savory egg patty and pairs it with spicy arugula, dressed simply in a light lemon vinaigrette.

DF
GF
NF
SF

SERVES 4 • PREP TIME: 10 minutes **• COOK TIME:** 30 minutes

2 teaspoons vegetable oil, divided

1 cup chopped fresh bean sprouts

3 scallions, chopped, white and green parts

1 small celery stalk, thinly sliced

1 teaspoon minced fresh ginger

6 eggs

1½ teaspoons salt, divided

1 tablespoon olive oil

1 teaspoon freshly squeezed lemon juice

2 cups arugula

TIP: Although you may be tempted to immediately transfer the hot vegetables to the beaten eggs, this may cause the eggs to start cooking. Ensuring your vegetables have slightly cooled will prevent this and also make for evenly cooked patties.

1 In a medium skillet over medium-high heat, heat 1 teaspoon vegetable oil until shimmering. Add the bean sprouts, scallions, celery, and ginger and sauté until tender, 4 to 5 minutes. Remove from the skillet and set aside to cool for 5 minutes.

2 In a large bowl, beat the eggs with 1 teaspoon salt. Add the cooled vegetable mixture and stir to combine.

3 Lower the heat to medium and add the remaining 1 teaspoon vegetable oil to the skillet. Pour in one-quarter of the egg mixture to form a small patty. Cook until golden brown on the bottom, 3 to 4 minutes. Flip and cook the other side until brown, about 3 more minutes.

4 Repeat three more times with the remaining egg mixture, adding more vegetable oil as needed.

5 In a medium bowl, combine the remaining ½ teaspoon salt with the olive oil and lemon juice to make a light vinaigrette. Add the arugula to the bowl and toss to coat.

6 Serve one-quarter of the dressed arugula over each egg foo young patty.

PER SERVING (¼ RECIPE): Calories: 167; Total fat: 13g; Protein: 10g; Total carbs: 4g; Fiber: 1g; Net carbs: 3g

MACROS: Fat: 70%; Protein: 24%; Carbs: 6%

Thai-Inspired Peanut Roasted Cauliflower

Peanut butter is a controversial keto food, because peanuts are a legume, but if you use a no-sugar-added brand or make your own, you can certainly enjoy it in moderation. This is another side dish that stands on its own as a light lunch or dinner.

SERVES 2 • PREP TIME: 10 minutes • **COOK TIME:** 20 minutes

½ head cauliflower, cut into bite-size florets

1 tablespoon olive oil

Salt

Freshly ground black pepper

½ cup unsweetened full-fat coconut milk

2 tablespoons sugar-free peanut butter

¼ teaspoon red curry paste

1 clove garlic, minced

1 tablespoon chopped fresh or dried parsley

1 Preheat the oven to 400°F.

2 On a baking sheet, arrange the cauliflower in a single layer. Drizzle with the olive oil and season with salt and pepper. Roast for 20 minutes or until the edges are brown.

3 While the cauliflower is cooking, in a blender, combine the coconut milk, peanut butter, curry paste, and garlic. Process until smooth.

4 Divide the cauliflower between two plates and drizzle the peanut sauce over top. Garnish with the parsley and serve.

PER SERVING (½ RECIPE): Calories: 290; Total fat: 27g; Protein: 8g; Total carbs: 9g; Fiber: 3g; Net carbs: 6g

MACROS: Fat: 84%; Protein: 11%; Carbs: 5%

Egg Cauliflower Tikka Masala

Tikka masala is a not-too-spicy curry dish with a creamy tomato-based sauce. Curry is a spice mixture—not a single spice—so not all curries taste the same. Traditional curry spices include cinnamon, cloves, coriander, cumin, ginger, paprika, and turmeric. You can also add a pinch of garam masala for an authentic taste.

SERVES 4 • PREP TIME: 15 minutes • **COOK TIME:** 35 minutes

2 tablespoons olive oil

1 white onion, chopped

2 teaspoons minced garlic

1 teaspoon grated
fresh ginger

1 head cauliflower, cut into
small florets

3 tablespoons red
curry paste

1 cup Vegetable Broth
(page 108) or store-bought
vegetable broth

8 large hard-boiled eggs,
peeled and halved
lengthwise

1 cup fresh baby spinach

2 cups heavy (whip-
ping) cream

2 tablespoons chopped
fresh cilantro, for garnish

1. In a large skillet over medium-high heat, heat the olive oil until shimmering. Add the onion, garlic, and ginger and sauté until softened, about 4 minutes. Add the cauliflower and curry paste and stir to coat.

2. Add the broth and bring to a boil. Reduce the heat to low and simmer, partially covered, until the vegetables are tender, about 20 minutes.

3. Add the eggs and spinach and simmer to heat through, about 6 minutes. Stir in the heavy cream and simmer for 2 minutes until warmed.

4. Serve topped with the cilantro.

TIP: To increase the protein, whisk 2 scoops of a low-carb unflavored protein powder into the cream before adding to the curry. This increases the calories to 718 and changes the macros to Fat: 75%; Protein: 19%; Carbs: 6%.

PER SERVING (¼ RECIPE): Calories: 668; Total fat: 60g; Protein: 18g; Total carbs: 14g; Fiber: 3g; Net carbs: 11g

MACROS: Fat: 80%; Protein: 12%; Carbs: 8%

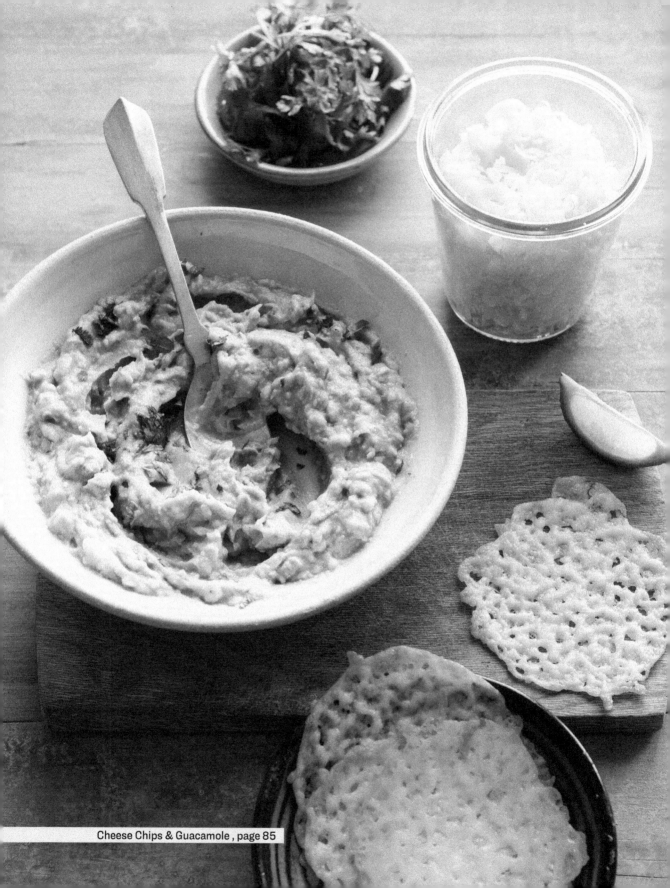

Cheese Chips & Guacamole , page 85

CHAPTER 6

Snacks

Zucchini Chips 5 GF OP SF V 84

Cheese Chips & Guacamole EF 5 GF NF Q SF 85

Parmesan Radishes EF 5 GF NF SF 86

Fondue and Crudités EF GF NF Q SF 87

Taco Tots and Dipping Sauce GF SF 88

Gourmet "Cheese" Balls GF V 90

Cookie Fat Bombs 5 GF SF V 91

Chili Chocolate Fat Bombs 5 GF Q SF V 92

Zucchini Chips

Salty and crunchy, these zucchini chips are light yet satisfying and a great go-to when hunger strikes. They're especially handy when you don't want to go over your macros for the day. Don't let the simplicity of this recipe fool you, either; the chips are a good source of vitamins C and A, thiamin, niacin, and fiber.

SERVES 6 • PREP TIME: 10 minutes **• COOK TIME:** 2 hours

1 large zucchini, cut into thin disks

1 teaspoon salt

2 tablespoons coconut oil, melted

1 teaspoon dried dill

1 tablespoon freshly ground black pepper

1 Preheat the oven to 225°F. Line a baking sheet with parchment paper or aluminum foil.

2 Spread the zucchini slices out on paper towels and sprinkle them with the salt. Let sit for 5 minutes. With a separate paper towel, firmly press the zucchini slices and pat them dry (the drier the better).

3 Transfer the zucchini slices to the baking sheet and toss with the coconut oil, dill, and pepper. Spread the slices into a single layer.

4 Bake for 2 hours or until golden and crisp. Check every 30 minutes or so to avoid burning. If you see them beginning to burn, remove the chips immediately.

5 Cool completely before transferring the chips to a serving bowl. Store leftovers in an airtight container for up to 3 days.

TIP: To create barbecue chips, toss the slices in your favorite barbecue rub and a few drops of liquid stevia before baking. Be sure not to oversalt them.

PER SERVING (⅙ RECIPE): Calories: 52; Total fat: 5g; Protein: 1g; Total carbs: 3g; Fiber: 1g; Net carbs: 2g

MACROS: Fat: 86%; Protein: 7%; Carbs: 7%

Cheese Chips & Guacamole

Chips and guacamole are one of those appetizers you miss when you are on a keto diet. But these cheese chips are so easy to make, there is no reason to miss chips. And you may even like these better. For an extra kick, add some of the diced jalapeños to the cheese mixture before baking the chips.

EF
5
GF
NF
Q
SF

SERVES 2 • PREP TIME: 10 minutes • **COOK TIME:** 7 minutes

1 cup shredded cheese (such as Mexican blend)

1 avocado, pitted, peeled, and mashed

2 tablespoons chopped fresh cilantro

Juice of ½ lime

1 teaspoon diced jalapeño pepper

Salt

Freshly ground black pepper

1. Preheat the oven to 350°F. Line a baking sheet with parchment paper or a silicone baking mat.

2. Make four ¼-cup mounds of shredded cheese on the prepared baking sheet, leaving plenty of space between them. Bake until the edges are brown and the middles have fully melted, about 7 minutes.

3. Set on a wire rack to cool for 5 minutes. The chips will be floppy when they first come out of the oven but will crisp as they cool.

4. In a medium bowl, mix together the avocado, cilantro, lime juice, and jalapeño to make the guacamole. Season with salt and pepper to taste.

5. Top the cheese chips evenly with guacamole and serve.

PER SERVING (2 CHIPS AND ½ THE GUACAMOLE): Calories: 323; Total fat: 27g; Protein: 15g; Total carbs: 8g; Fiber: 5g; Net carbs: 3g

MACROS: Fat: 75%; Protein: 18%; Carbs: 7%

Parmesan Radishes

Ghee is the culinary term for clarified butter, which you can purchase by the jar at the grocery store. The casein and lactose (dairy solids) are removed from butter, leaving clear, liquid fat. Ghee's high smoke point makes it ideal for roasting and high-temperature cooking.

SERVES 2 • PREP TIME: 10 minutes • **COOK TIME:** 35 minutes

12 radishes, trimmed and quartered

2 tablespoons ghee, melted

1 teaspoon fresh thyme leaves

½ teaspoon salt

2 tablespoons grated vegetarian Parmesan

1 Preheat the oven to 400°F. Line a baking sheet with parchment paper.

2 In a medium bowl, coat the radishes in the melted ghee. Season with the thyme and salt.

3 Place the radishes on the baking sheet and bake for 30 minutes, until tender. Sprinkle with the Parmesan and bake for another 3 to 5 minutes until the cheese is melted and golden.

TIP: To make this dish vegan, use vegan Parmesan (or omit it) and substitute vegetable ghee. Otherwise known as vegetable shortening, vegetable ghee is primarily composed of vegetable oil and is naturally dairy-free.

PER SERVING (½ RECIPE): Calories: 143; Total fat: 15g; Protein: 2g; Total carbs: 2g; Fiber: 1g; Net carbs: 1g

MACROS: Fat: 94%; Protein: 5%; Carbs: 1%

Fondue and Crudités

EF

GF

NF

Q

SF

When my husband and I started dating, he would take me to La Fondue in Saratoga, California, every Valentine's Day for a fondue feast. Little did I know that years later, fondue would become one of my favorite keto indulgences. There's something about pickles and cheese that makes me forget all about the cubes of bread—plus, they stay on the fork more easily.

SERVES 2 • PREP TIME: 15 minutes • **COOK TIME:** 15 minutes

¼ pound Swiss cheese, grated

¼ pound white cheddar, grated

1 teaspoon xanthan gum

1 cup dry white wine (such as Chardonnay or Sauvignon Blanc)

½ teaspoon minced garlic

½ teaspoon freshly squeezed lemon juice

4 gherkin pickles, halved

8 radishes, trimmed and quartered

1 cup thinly sliced fennel

1 bell pepper, any color, sliced

1 In a large bowl, toss the grated cheeses with the xanthan gum until evenly distributed. Set aside.

2 In a large pot over medium-low heat, combine the wine, garlic, and lemon juice. Bring to a simmer, then add the cheeses a few tablespoons at a time, stirring constantly, until completed melted and smooth.

3 Transfer the fondue to a serving bowl and serve alongside the gherkins, radishes, fennel, and bell pepper for dipping.

TIP: If you don't have any lemons on hand, substitute ½ teaspoon of Dijon or brown mustard for some mellow heat.

PER SERVING (½ RECIPE): Calories: 643; Total fat: 38g; Protein: 32g; Total carbs: 24g; Fiber: 4g; Net carbs: 20g

MACROS: Fat: 53%; Protein: 20%; Carbs: 27%

Taco Tots and Dipping Sauce

Many of us fell in love with Tater Tots as children, but unfortunately, they are full of carbohydrates and contain an unhealthy amount of saturated fat that can raise cholesterol. Once I started making my own tots, I experimented with different combinations of vegetables. My research revealed that dense vegetables such as cauliflower, parsnips, and turnips make the best tots—but you can include colorful vegetables such as spinach, red peppers, and even purple cabbage to make the color of your tots pop. These tots are packed with taco-inspired flavor and are a cinch to make.

MAKES 24 TOTS • PREP TIME: 15 minutes • **COOK TIME:** 1 hour

2 cups peeled and diced turnips (from 3 medium turnips)

1 cup small cauliflower florets

1 tablespoon olive oil

1 slice Basic Bread (page 117) or store-bought keto bread, cubed

2 cups shredded white cheddar cheese

1 large egg, beaten

1 tablespoon plus 1 teaspoon sugar-free taco seasoning, divided

Salt (optional)

½ cup mayonnaise

1 teaspoon freshly squeezed lime juice

1 Preheat the oven to 400°F. Line two baking sheets with parchment paper.

2 On one of the baking sheets, toss the turnips and cauliflower in the olive oil. Roast for 15 minutes, then remove the baking sheet from the oven, create some space at either end, and add the cubed bread. Return the baking sheet to the oven and roast for 15 more minutes until the vegetables are tender and the bread is crisp. Set aside to cool for 5 minutes. Keep the oven on.

3 In a food processor, pulse the toasted bread a few times to create bread crumbs. Add the roasted turnips and cauliflower, along with the cheddar, egg, and 1 tablespoon taco seasoning. Pulse until the mixture forms a paste.

4 Using your hands, roll about 1 tablespoon of mixture into the shape of a Tater Tot and place on the second baking sheet. Repeat with the remaining tot mixture.

5 Bake for 30 minutes, until the tots are golden. Sprinkle them with salt, if desired.

6 In a small bowl, combine the remaining 1 teaspoon taco seasoning, mayonnaise, and lime juice. Serve the tots with the sauce for dipping.

TIP: For an Italian spin, replace 1 tablespoon taco seasoning with Italian seasoning, use shredded mozzarella instead of cheddar, and serve with marinara as your dipping sauce. Don't have turnips? Experiment with broccoli. No taco seasoning? A pinch of cumin and chili powder goes a long way. Prefer Indian flavors? Swap taco seasoning with a curry spice blend and add some shredded carrot.

PER SERVING (4 TOTS): Calories: 364; Total fat: 32g; Protein: 12g; Total carbs: 8g; Fiber: 2g; Net carbs: 6g

MACROS: Fat: 79%; Protein: 13%; Carbs: 8%

Gourmet "Cheese" Balls

Cheese lovers will gobble up these savory treats, and they may not even realize there's no cheese in the recipe. These "cheese" balls are high in fat and protein with an umami goodness that will curb even the unruli-est of appetites. You might want to make a double quantity of this recipe because they have a tendency to disappear fast.

MAKES 24 • PREP TIME: 20 minutes, plus overnight to soak and 1 hour to chill

1 cup raw hazelnuts, soaked overnight

¼ cup water

2 tablespoons nutri-tional yeast

1 teaspoon apple cider vinegar

1 teaspoon miso paste

1 teaspoon mustard

½ cup almond flour

1 cup slivered almonds

1 teaspoon dried oregano

1 In a blender, combine the hazelnuts, water, nutri-tional yeast, vinegar, miso paste, and mustard. Blend until well combined, thick, and creamy. Transfer the mixture to a medium bowl.

2 Slowly stir in the almond flour until the mixture forms a dough. Set aside.

3 In a small bowl, toss the almonds and oregano together. Set aside.

4 Scoop the hazelnut mixture by the tablespoon and use your hands to roll it into bite-size balls. Place the balls on a baking sheet. (You should have about 24 balls.)

5 One by one, roll the hazelnut balls in the almond and oregano mixture until thoroughly coated, and place back on the baking sheet.

6 Place the sheet in the refrigerator for 1 hour to chill before serving.

TIP: These can be made in advance and stored in an airtight container in the refrigerator for up to 1 week. Freezing is not recommended, as it will alter the texture.

PER SERVING (1 CHEESE BALL): Calories: 78; Total fat: 7g; Protein: 3g; Total carbs: 3g; Fiber: 2g; Net carbs: 1g

MACROS: Fat: 81%; Protein: 15%; Carbs: 4%

Cookie Fat Bombs

Fat bombs are the perfect pick-me-up between meals. These little balls of magic are high fat, low carb, and utterly delicious, making them the perfect snack or light dessert. Keep them on hand to satisfy sudden sugar cravings. They're also great for a pre-workout energy boost.

MAKES 12 • PREP TIME: 10 minutes, plus 40 minutes to chill

1 cup almond butter

½ cup coconut flour

1 teaspoon ground cinnamon

¼ cup cacao nibs or vegan keto chocolate chips

1 Line a baking sheet with parchment paper or aluminum foil.

2 In a bowl, whisk together the almond butter, coconut flour, and cinnamon. Fold in the cacao nibs.

3 Cover the bowl and chill in the freezer for 15 to 20 minutes.

4 Scoop the mixture by the tablespoon and roll between your palms to form a ball. Place it on the prepared baking sheet. Repeat to use all the mixture.

5 Chill in the freezer for 20 minutes until firm.

6 Store in an airtight container in the refrigerator for up to 2 weeks.

PER SERVING (1 FAT BOMB): Calories: 164; Total fat: 13g; Protein: 5g; Total carbs: 7g; Fiber: 4g; Net carbs: 3g

MACROS: Fat: 71%; Protein: 12%; Carbs: 17%

Chili Chocolate Fat Bombs

5

GF

Q

SF

V

Good-quality cocoa powder is an acceptable ingredient on the keto diet, which means you can still enjoy a chocolate snack when you need a fix. Dark chocolate like cocoa is very high in manganese, magnesium, copper, iron, and fiber, as well as antioxidants, which fight free radicals in the body. Dark chocolate has been found to help lower blood pressure, reduce cholesterol, and improve cognitive function.

MAKES 12 • PREP TIME: 10 minutes, plus 15 minutes to chill • **COOK TIME:** 5 minutes

¾ cup coconut oil

¼ cup cocoa powder

¼ cup almond butter

⅛ teaspoon chili powder

3 drops liquid stevia

1 Line the cups of a mini muffin tin with paper liners and set aside.

2 In a small saucepan over low heat, combine all the ingredients. Heat until the coconut oil is melted, about 4 minutes, then whisk to blend.

3 Spoon the mixture into the muffin cups and place the tin in the refrigerator until the bombs are firm, about 15 minutes.

4 Transfer the bombs to an airtight container and store in the freezer until you want to serve them.

PER SERVING (1 FAT BOMB): Calories: 117; Total fat: 12g; Protein: 2g; Total carbs: 2g; Fiber: 0g; Net carbs: 2g

MACROS: Fat: 92%; Protein: 7%; Carbs: 1%

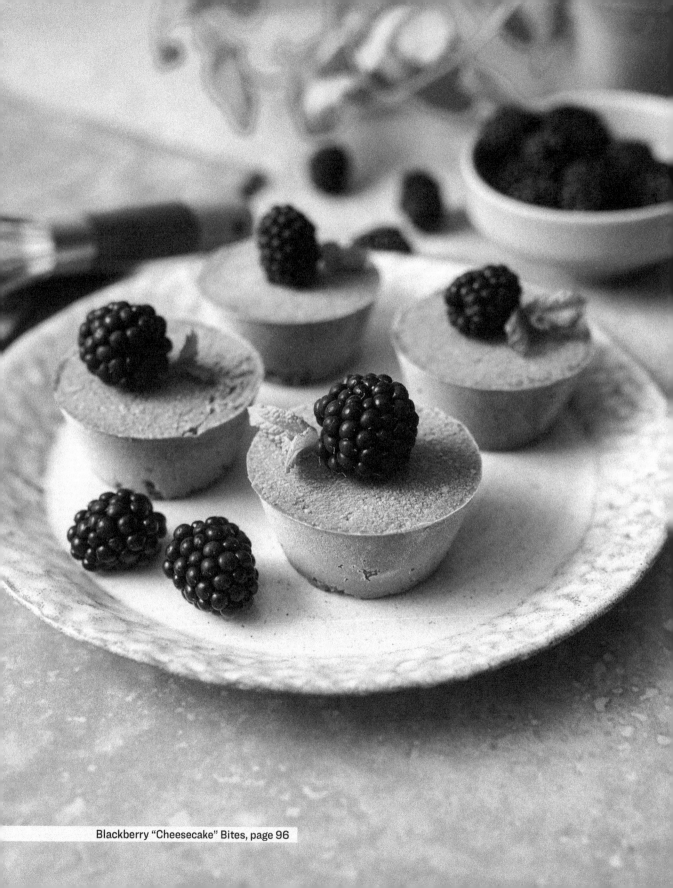

Blackberry "Cheesecake" Bites, page 96

CHAPTER 7

Desserts

Blackberry "Cheesecake" Bites GF SF V 96

Vanilla Pudding 5 GF NF OP SF 97

Chocolate Avocado Pudding 5 GF OP Q SF V 98

Raspberry Ice Cream EF 5 GF NF SF 99

Peanut Butter Cookies DF 5 GF Q SF 100

Pumpkin Spice Cookies GF Q SF 101

Carrot (Pan)Cake GF Q SF 102

Berry Cobbler DF GF SF 104

Blackberry "Cheesecake" Bites

That famous cheesecake restaurant doesn't have a thing on this dessert. These satisfying bites are so much healthier with the fat from the coconut, protein from the almonds, and antioxidants from the blackberries. Not to mention the sugar-free sweetness. It's a one-two-three-four power punch. Who says cheesecake isn't good for you?

SERVES 4 • PREP TIME: 1 hour 35 minutes, plus overnight to soak

1½ cups almonds, soaked overnight

1 cup fresh blackberries

⅓ cup coconut oil, melted

⅓ cup allulose

¼ cup full-fat coconut cream

¼ cup freshly squeezed lemon juice

1 Line the cups of a 12-cup muffin tin with cupcake liners.

2 In a blender, combine all the ingredients. Blend on high until the mixture is whipped and fluffy.

3 Divide the mixture equally among the muffin cups.

4 Place the muffin tin in the freezer for 1 hour, 30 minutes to allow the cheesecake bites to set. Serve cold.

TIP: This dessert is wonderful for preparing ahead, particularly for special occasions, because you can keep it in the freezer. To thaw, place the bites on the countertop for 1 hour to come to room temperature.

PER SERVING (3 BITES): Calories: 514; Total fat: 48g; Protein: 12g; Total carbs: 18g; Fiber: 9g; Net carbs: 9g

MACROS: Fat: 84%; Protein: 9%; Carbs: 7%

Vanilla Pudding

Pudding from scratch? You can do it. This recipe is a base that you can adapt in countless ways to satisfy your every craving. Like an extra-silky pudding? Whisk in a tablespoon of butter as the pudding cooks for a velvety smooth texture.

5
GF
NF
OP
SF

SERVES 2 • PREP TIME: 5 minutes, plus 1 hour to chill • **COOK TIME:** 10 minutes

1 cup cream

3 egg yolks

3 tablespoons erythritol

½ teaspoon vanilla extract

1 In a medium saucepan over medium-low heat, whisk together the cream, egg yolks, and erythritol. Whisk gently every 1 to 2 minutes until the mixture is bubbling and thick, about 10 minutes total.

2 Remove from the heat and stir in the vanilla.

3 Chill in the refrigerator for at least 1 hour before serving.

TIP: How about a pudding party? Make a few batches of the vanilla pudding base and invite your guests to get creative with keto-friendly mix-ins, like chopped pistachios, mashed strawberries, and toasted coconut.

PER SERVING (½ RECIPE): Calories: 478; Total fat: 49g; Protein: 7g; Total carbs: 22g; Fiber: 0g; Net carbs: 4g

MACROS: Fat: 92%; Protein: 6%; Carbs: 2%

Chocolate Avocado Pudding

Avocados make the creamiest, most delicious puddings. They have a neutral flavor that can be easily blended with other flavors such as chocolate or cinnamon. This recipe will quickly become a weekly, if not daily, staple for your ketogenic diet.

SERVES 1 · PREP TIME: 5 minutes

1 avocado, halved

⅓ cup unsweetened full-fat coconut milk

2 tablespoons unsweetened cocoa powder

1 teaspoon vanilla extract

5 or 6 drops liquid stevia

In a blender or food processor, combine all the ingredients and blend until smooth. Serve immediately.

TIP: For an ice cream–type treat, place the pudding in the freezer for 20 minutes or until it reaches a soft-serve consistency.

PER SERVING (ENTIRE RECIPE): Calories: 555; Total fat: 47g; Protein: 7g; Total carbs: 26g; Fiber: 17g; Net carbs: 9g

MACROS: Fat: 76%; Protein: 5%; Carbs: 19%

Raspberry Ice Cream

EF

5

GF

NF

SF

Strawberries were my berry of choice until I learned that raspberries are 25 percent lower in carbohydrates, contain more fiber, and are loaded with flavonoids (phytonutrients that kick-start your immune system and flush away toxins).

SERVES 2 • PREP TIME: 10 minutes, plus 4 to 6 hours to chill

12 raspberries

1½ cups heavy (whipping) cream

1 cup cream cheese, at room temperature

¼ cup erythritol

2 tablespoons freshly squeezed lemon juice

1 In a blender, combine the raspberries and cream. Blend until pureed.

2 Transfer to a glass bowl and stir in the cream cheese, erythritol, and lemon juice.

3 Freeze for 4 to 6 hours until frozen but scoopable.

TIP: If you don't have any lemons, reduce the heavy cream measurement to 1¼ cups and add ¼ cup of full-fat sour cream.

PER SERVING (½ RECIPE): Calories: 1022; Total fat: 105g; Protein: 12g; Total carbs: 38g; Fiber: 1g; Net carbs: 13g

MACROS: Fat: 92%; Protein: 5%; Carbs: 3%

Peanut Butter Cookies

You can't beat the crumbly, nutty sweetness of peanut butter cookies, and these dairy-free keto ones don't disappoint. For extra indulgence, top them with a few keto-friendly dark chocolate chips just before putting them into the oven.

MAKES ABOUT 15 COOKIES • PREP TIME: 15 minutes • **COOK TIME:** 15 minutes

1 cup powdered sugar alternative (such as Swerve)

¾ cup sugar-free peanut butter

¼ cup olive oil

1 large egg

1 Preheat the oven to 325°F. Line a baking sheet with parchment paper.

2 In a medium bowl, combine all the ingredients and mix well.

3 Roll the dough into 1-inch balls and arrange them on the prepared baking sheet 2 inches apart. Press the tines of a fork into each cookie to get the traditional crosshatch design.

4 Bake for 12 minutes or until lightly browned and crisp. Cool for 5 minutes in the pan before serving warm, or transfer to a wire rack to cool completely.

PER SERVING (1 COOKIE): Calories: 118; Total fat: 10g; Protein: 4g; Total carbs: 3g; Fiber: 1g; Net carbs: 2g

MACROS: Fat: 76%; Protein: 14%; Carbs: 10%

Pumpkin Spice Cookies

GF

Q

SF

My keto desserts took a deliciously splendid turn when I discovered nut flours. You can purchase them pre-ground in a very fine, dustlike consistency; however, it's much more affordable (and somewhat therapeutic) to pulverize your own nuts. Pecans work very well for this recipe—pumpkin pie spices and pecans evoke a lovely holiday sentiment—but hazelnuts or walnuts work just as beautifully. When I am running low on pumpkin pie spice, I substitute apple pie spice, which offers the same warm notes, with a touch of cardamom.

MAKES 10 COOKIES • PREP TIME: 10 minutes • **COOK TIME:** 15 minutes

2 cups chopped pecans

1 egg, beaten

½ cup unsalted butter, at room temperature

¼ cup erythritol

1 tablespoon pumpkin pie spice

1 teaspoon vanilla extract

Nonstick cooking spray

1 Preheat the oven to 350°F. Line a baking sheet with parchment paper.

2 Place the pecans in a sealable plastic bag. Using a mallet or the back of a large spoon, crush the nuts until they become flour-like in consistency with no large pieces of pecan.

3 Transfer the pecan flour to a medium bowl and add the egg, butter, erythritol, pumpkin pie spice, and vanilla. Mix to form a cohesive dough.

4 Roll the dough into 1-inch balls and space them out on the baking sheet. You should have about 10 cookies total. Coat the bottom of a glass with a thin layer of cooking spray and use it to flatten the dough into circles.

5 Bake the cookies for 12 to 15 minutes, until the edges begin to brown.

6 Cool for 5 minutes on the sheet, then transfer to a wire rack to cool for another 5 to 10 minutes until firm.

TIP: Make your own pumpkin pie spice from 4 parts ground cinnamon, 2 parts ground ginger, 1 part ground cloves, and 1 part ground nutmeg.

PER SERVING (2 COOKIES): Calories: 484; Total fat: 51g; Protein: 5g; Total carbs: 17g; Fiber: 4g; Net carbs: 3g

MACROS: Fat: 95%; Protein: 4%; Carbs: 1%

Carrot (Pan)Cake

I don't consider myself a highly skilled baker, which is why I like to make (pan)cake desserts. No oven needed—just two low-carb, warmly spiced pancakes, cooked on the stove, slathered in slightly more frosting than you really need. Because bleached flour, or all-purpose flour, is rich in carbohydrates, I substitute pulverized walnuts. Walnut "flour" adds a depth of flavor and complements the sweetness of the carrots to create a perfectly balanced "cake" with a fraction of the effort.

SERVES 2 • PREP TIME: 10 minutes **• COOK TIME:** 10 minutes

FOR THE CARROT CAKE

1 cup chopped walnuts

1 tablespoon pumpkin
   pie spice

1 teaspoon baking powder

1 teaspoon erythritol

½ cup shredded carrot

1 egg, beaten

3 tablespoons half-and-half

2 tablespoons melted butter

Pinch salt

TO MAKE THE CARROT CAKE

1 Place the walnuts in a sealable plastic bag. Using a mallet or the back of a large spoon, crush the walnuts until they become flour-like in consistency with no large pieces of walnut.

2 Transfer the walnut flour to a medium bowl and add the pumpkin pie spice, baking powder, and erythritol. Stir to combine.

3 To the same bowl, add the carrot, egg, half-and-half, butter, and salt. Stir until just combined.

4 Set a nonstick skillet over medium-low heat. Once hot, add half the batter and cook for 2 to 3 minutes, until brown on the bottom. Flip and cook for an additional 1 to 2 minutes, until the interior of the cake is completely cooked (test with a toothpick if needed). Transfer the cake to a plate and repeat with the remaining batter.

FOR THE FROSTING

4 ounces cream cheese, at room temperature

2 tablespoons half-and-half

1 teaspoon vanilla extract

TO MAKE THE FROSTING

5 In a small bowl, combine the cream cheese, half-and-half, and vanilla and mix until smooth.

6 Frost one cake layer with half the frosting. Place the second cake layer on top and cover with the remaining frosting.

TIP: The cake batter is thick and can be a little challenging to work with. Feel free to reduce the heat to low if the cake starts to brown too quickly.

PER SERVING (½ RECIPE): Calories: 794; Total fat: 76g; Protein: 17g; Total carbs: 21g; Fiber: 5g; Net carbs: 14g

MACROS: Fat: 86%; Protein: 9%; Carbs: 5%

Berry Cobbler

Who doesn't love a good cobbler with ice cream? Unfortunately, a good cobbler with ice cream isn't keto-friendly. Enter: this recipe, which swaps in coconut milk, coconut oil, and almond flour. (Always remember to eat berries in moderation only.)

SERVES 6 • PREP TIME: 10 minutes • **COOK TIME:** 30 minutes

1 pint fresh blueberries

½ pint fresh blackberries

1 cup erythritol, divided

¼ cup unsweetened full-fat coconut milk

½ cup coconut oil

1 large egg

1 teaspoon vanilla extract

½ cup almond flour

1 teaspoon salt

1 teaspoon baking powder

1 Preheat the oven to 350°F.

2 In a 9-inch square baking dish, toss together the blueberries, blackberries, ¼ cup erythritol, and the coconut milk.

3 In a microwave-safe bowl, melt the coconut oil until liquefied, about 2 minutes. Add ¼ cup erythritol, the egg, and vanilla and whisk until well blended.

4 In another small bowl, combine the remaining ½ cup erythritol with the almond flour, salt, and baking powder. Add the dry ingredients to the egg mixture and mix to combine.

5 Dollop spoonfuls of the crust mixture over the berry mixture in the baking dish.

6 Bake for 30 minutes or until browned on top. Serve hot.

PER SERVING (⅙ RECIPE): Calories: 241; Total fat: 22g; Protein: 2g; Total carbs: 10g; Fiber: 3g; Net carbs: 7g

MACROS: Fat: 81%; Protein: 4%; Carbs: 15%

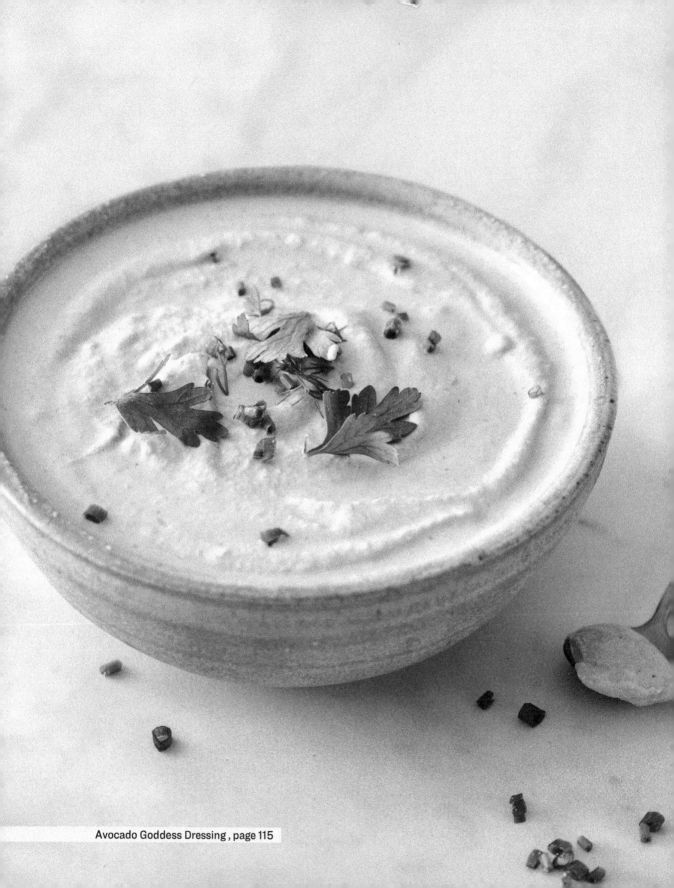

Avocado Goddess Dressing , page 115

CHAPTER 8

Homemade Staples

Vegetable Broth GF NF SF V 108

Madeline's Marinade 5 GF NF OP Q SF V 109

Classic Pesto EF 5 GF OP Q SF 110

Pico de Gallo 5 GF NF OP Q SF V 111

Chimichurri 5 GF NF OP Q SF V 112

Bagna Cauda Dip EF 5 NF OP Q 113

Balsamic Vinaigrette 5 GF NF OP Q SF V 114

Avocado Goddess Dressing GF NF OP Q SF V 115

Ranch Dressing GF NF OP Q SF 116

Basic Bread 5 GF Q SF 117

Vegan Eggs, Two Ways 5 GF NF OP Q SF V 118

Tempeh "Bacon" GF NF Q V 119

Vegetable Broth

Just about any combination of aromatics, herbs, and vegetables will create a rich broth that you can use for soups and stews. A tablespoon of vegetable broth is a lifesaver for vegetables that are overly roasted, a cheese sauce that's a little too thick, or mashed cauliflower that needs a flavor boost.

MAKES 12 CUPS • PREP TIME: 10 minutes • COOK TIME: 35 minutes

1 cup sliced leeks

1 cup diced carrots

½ cup sliced celery

5 Italian parsley sprigs

2 thyme sprigs

2 rosemary sprigs

1 bay leaf

1 teaspoon salt

1 teaspoon freshly ground black pepper

3 quarts water

1 In a large pot over high heat, combine all the ingredients.

2 Bring to a boil, then reduce the heat to medium-low. Simmer for about 30 minutes to develop the flavors.

3 Remove from the heat and cool completely, then strain through a fine-mesh sieve.

4 Refrigerate in airtight containers for up to a week or freeze in ice cube trays for up to 3 months.

TIP: Don't throw away the vegetables after making this broth. Put them in a food processor with a pinch of salt, 1 cup of frozen (thawed) peas, and 1 tablespoon of almond flour to make veggie burgers. Panfry in olive oil over medium heat for 3 for 5 minutes per side.

PER SERVING (1 CUP): Calories: 5; Total fat: 0g; Protein: <1g; Total carbs: 1g; Fiber: <1g; Net carbs: <1g

MACROS: Fat: 0%; Protein: 0%; Carbs: 100%

Madeline's Marinade

My grandmother, Madeline, created this marinade many years ago to infuse flavor into inexpensive cuts of meat. It's equally as delicious when paired with "meaty" vegetables such as portabella mushrooms, asparagus, and even cauliflower steaks.

MAKES 1 CUP • PREP TIME: 5 minutes

½ cup olive oil

½ cup red wine vinegar

4 cloves garlic, crushed

3 tablespoons chopped fresh rosemary

2 teaspoons salt

1 teaspoon freshly ground black pepper

In a small bowl, combine all the ingredients. Cover 4 cups of diced vegetables of your choice with the marinade and refrigerate for at least 1 hour to achieve maximum flavor.

TIP: When you need a quick, creamy salad dressing, combine 1 tablespoon of mayonnaise for every 2 tablespoons of marinade.

PER SERVING (¼ CUP): Calories: 252; Total fat: 28g; Protein: 1g; Total carbs: 2g; Fiber: 1g; Net carbs: 1g

MACROS: Fat: 98%; Protein: 1%; Carbs: 1%

Classic Pesto

Pesto is derived from the Italian verb pestare *("to pound or crush"). This recipe features the classic Genoese version, but I encourage you to adapt it to your taste. Try arugula instead of basil, or hazelnuts instead of pine nuts.*

MAKES 1 CUP • PREP TIME: 5 minutes

1 cup fresh basil

½ cup grated vegetarian
Parmesan cheese

¼ cup pine nuts

2 cloves garlic

⅔ cup extra-virgin olive oil

1 In a food processor, combine the basil, Parmesan, pine nuts, and garlic. Process until a thick paste forms.

2 With the motor running, slowly drizzle in the olive oil until the pesto reaches your desired consistency.

TIP: When pesto appears in a dish, it's often the main attraction; however, that doesn't mean it can't play a supporting role. Add pesto to mayonnaise, mashed cauliflower, or scrambled eggs for freshness and flavor.

PER SERVING (2 TABLESPOONS): Calories: 214;
Total fat: 23g; Protein: 3g; Total carbs: 2g; Fiber: <1g;
Net carbs: <1g

MACROS: Fat: 96%; Protein: 4%; Carbs: 0%

Pico de Gallo

My favorite pico de gallo preparation has equal parts diced tomato and onion, with a little jalapeño for heat. Because the acid from the lime juice immediately begins to break down the vegetables, remove the tomato seeds and pulp prior to dicing to prevent excess liquid from collecting in the bottom of the bowl.

MAKES 2 CUPS • PREP TIME: 10 minutes, plus 20 minutes to marinate

¾ cup diced white onion

¾ cup seeded and diced Roma tomatoes (about 4)

½ cup chopped fresh cilantro

3 tablespoons freshly squeezed lime juice

1 tablespoon minced jalapeño pepper

1 teaspoon salt

In a small bowl, combine all the ingredients. Allow the flavors to develop for 15 to 20 minutes before serving.

TIP: Try to consume pico de gallo as soon as possible after the flavors meld, because raw onion is a magnet for bacteria, even when stored in an airtight container.

PER SERVING (¼ CUP): Calories: 8; Total fat: 0g; Protein: <1g; Total carbs: 2g; Fiber: 1g; Net carbs: 1g

MACROS: Fat: 0%; Protein: <1% Carbs: 99%

Chimichurri

The red chile peppers found in chimichurri are often labeled "Fresno chiles" in the grocery store. Similar in size to jalapeños, they are a bit fruitier and spicier, which makes for a great balance in this herbaceous and acidic Argentinian condiment.

10 TABLESPOONS · PREP TIME: 10 minutes, plus 20 minutes to marinate

1 cup minced fresh Italian parsley

⅓ cup olive oil

¼ cup red wine vinegar

1 medium red chile, minced

2 cloves garlic, minced

1 teaspoon dried oregano

½ teaspoon salt

In a small bowl, combine all the ingredients. Allow the flavors to develop for 15 to 20 minutes before serving. Refrigerate leftovers in an airtight container for up to 10 days.

TIP: Chimichurri is a raw sauce; however, it's also scrumptious in sautés and as a flavor boost for canned vegetable soup.

PER SERVING (2 TABLESPOONS): Calories: 135; Total fat: 14g; Protein: 1g; Total carbs: 1g; Fiber: 1g; Net carbs: <1g

MACROS: Fat: 93%; Protein: 7%; Carbs: <1%

Bagna Cauda Dip

Traditionally made with anchovies, this Northern Italian dip is served warm with vegetables. The substitution of soy sauce for anchovies guarantees the saltiness isn't lost—a must for crudités such as celery and radishes.

MAKES 1 CUP • PREP TIME: 5 minutes • **COOK TIME:** 10 minutes

5 tablespoons butter

½ cup sour cream

2 tablespoons soy sauce

1 tablespoon minced garlic

1 In a small saucepan over low heat, melt the butter. Add the sour cream, soy sauce, and garlic and stir gently until the dip is well combined.

2 Simmer for about 5 minutes, until thickened. Serve with your favorite vegetable dippers.

TIP: If you're not a fan of sour cream, try a little Greek yogurt instead. Generally milder in flavor, yogurt will deliver the creaminess needed to balance the sharpness of the garlic.

PER SERVING (2 TABLESPOONS): Calories: 96; Total fat: 10g; Protein: 1g; Total carbs: 1g; Fiber: 0g; Net carbs: 1g

MACROS: Fat: 94%; Protein: 4%; Carbs: 2%

Balsamic Vinaigrette

The cost of balsamic vinegar varies wildly due to age, region, and purity. Although expensive, thick balsamic vinegars are delicious when drizzled on fruit. For this vinaigrette, an inexpensive balsamic is perfectly acceptable.

MAKES 1 CUP • PREP TIME: 5 minutes

¾ cup extra-virgin olive oil

¼ cup balsamic vinegar

1 tablespoon Dijon mustard

1 teaspoon minced garlic

½ teaspoon salt

½ teaspoon freshly ground black pepper

In a small bowl, combine all the ingredients and whisk until well incorporated.

TIP: White balsamic vinegar is often more affordable than its dark brown counterpart because it is aged for less than a year to retain its pale hue.

PER SERVING (2 TABLESPOONS): Calories: 189; Total fat: 20g; Protein: <1g; Total carbs: 2g; Fiber: <1g; Net carbs: 2g

MACROS: Fat: 95%; Protein: <1%; Carbs: 5%

Avocado Goddess Dressing

The traditional version of green goddess dressing contains anchovy, mayonnaise, and sour cream. My version is vividly vegan by omitting all those ingredients and substituting creamy, rich avocado. Apple cider vinegar gives this version a pop of acidity, while preserving its herbaceous character.

GF
NF
OP
Q
SF
V

MAKES 2 CUPS • PREP TIME: 10 minutes

2 medium avocados, peeled and pitted

½ cup chopped fresh cilantro

½ cup chopped fresh parsley

¼ cup chopped scallions, white and green parts

¼ cup extra-virgin olive oil

2 tablespoons freshly squeezed lemon juice

2 tablespoons apple cider vinegar

1 teaspoon minced garlic

1 teaspoon salt

Water (optional)

In a food processor, combine all the ingredients except the water and blend until smooth. Add water 1 tablespoon at a time as needed to reach your desired consistency.

TIP: If you choose not to add any water, this dressing is the perfect consistency for a dip.

PER SERVING (¼ CUP): Calories: 121; Total fat: 12g; Protein: 1g; Total carbs: 4g; Fiber: 3g; Net carbs: 1g

MACROS: Fat: 89%; Protein: 3%; Carbs: 8%

Ranch Dressing

This classic is great as a dip for vegetables, and of course as a dressing for green salads. It's really easy to make at home, which helps you cut down on the amount of preservatives you consume. If you want, make a big batch of the spice mix so it's ready to go when you need it (the spice mix is also great for seasoning vegetables before grilling).

MAKES ABOUT 1½ CUPS • PREP TIME: 5 minutes

1 cup mayonnaise

½ cup sour cream

1½ teaspoons dried chives

1 teaspoon mustard powder

½ teaspoon dried dill

½ teaspoon celery seed

½ teaspoon onion powder

½ teaspoon garlic powder

Salt

Freshly ground black pepper

In a medium bowl, combine the mayonnaise, sour cream, chives, mustard powder, dill, celery seed, onion powder, and garlic powder. Season with salt and pepper. Stir well to combine and refrigerate in an airtight container with a lid until ready to use. This will keep in the refrigerator for about 1 week.

PER SERVING (2 TABLESPOONS): Calories: 43; Total fat: 3g; Protein: 1g; Total carbs: 3g; Fiber: 1g; Net carbs: 2g

MACROS: Fat: 63%; Protein: 9%; Carbs: 28%

Basic Bread

There are lots of keto-friendly bread variations out there, but this one has a wonderful texture and works as a great basic recipe for creating sweet or savory variations. You don't have to use the MCT oil, but it is flavorless and adds high-quality fats.

SERVES 12 (MAKES 1 LOAF) • **PREP TIME:** 5 minutes • **COOK TIME:** 25 minutes

5 tablespoons unsalted butter, at room temperature, divided

6 large eggs, lightly beaten

1½ cups almond flour

3 teaspoons baking powder

1 scoop MCT oil powder (optional)

Pinch salt

1. Preheat the oven to 390°F. Grease a 9-by-5-inch loaf pan with 1 tablespoon butter.

2. In a large bowl, use an electric handheld mixer on medium speed to combine the eggs, almond flour, remaining 4 tablespoons butter, baking powder, MCT oil powder (if using), and salt until thoroughly blended. Pour into the prepared pan.

3. Bake for 25 minutes or until a toothpick inserted into the center of the loaf comes out clean.

4. Cool completely on a wire rack before slicing and serving.

PUMPKIN BREAD VARIATION

In step 2, add ¼ can of pure pumpkin puree (not pumpkin pie filling, which contains sugar), 2 to 3 teaspoons of liquid stevia (depending on how sweet you want it), and 1 tablespoon of pumpkin pie spice along with the other ingredients. Continue with the recipe as written.

CHOCOLATE CHIP BREAD VARIATION

Just before transferring to the loaf pan, fold ½ cup of keto-friendly chocolate chips (such as Lily's brand) into the batter. Continue with the recipe as written.

PER SERVING (1 SLICE): Calories: 165; Total fat: 15g; Protein: 6g; Total carbs: 4g; Fiber: 2g; Net carbs: 2g

MACROS: Fat: 82%; Protein: 14%; Carbs: 4%

Vegan Eggs, Two Ways

There are a couple of clever ways to replace eggs using plant-based sources. Flax and chia seeds are perfect for binding cakes, cookies, and bread. Aquafaba is the clever name for something surprising: the liquid from canned chickpeas. Best known as an egg white replacement, it also works to bind ingredients together and can act as a substitute for oil.

MAKES 1 EGG • PREP TIME: 5 to 10 minutes

FOR THE FLAX OR CHIA EGG

3 tablespoons warm water (90° to 110°F)

1 tablespoon ground flax-seed or chia seeds

FOR THE AQUAFABA EGG

3 tablespoons aquafaba

TO MAKE THE FLAX OR CHIA EGG

In a small bowl or measuring cup, whisk together 3 tablespoons warm water and 1 tablespoon ground flaxseed (or chia seeds) for each egg called for in the recipe. Let stand for 10 minutes to thicken before using.

TO MAKE THE AQUAFABA EGG

Drain the liquid from a can of chickpeas and set aside 3 tablespoons for each egg called for in the recipe. Store any remaining aquafaba for later use (see tip).

FLAXSEED PER SERVING (1 EGG): Calories: 37; Total fat: 3g; Protein: 1g; Total carbs: 2g; Fiber: 2g; Net carbs: 0g

MACROS: Fat: 73%; Protein: 11%; Carbs: 16%

CHIA SEED PER SERVING (1 EGG): Calories: 69; Total Fat: 4g; Protein: 2g; Total carbs: 6g; Fiber: 5g; Net carbs: 1g

MACROS: Fat: 52%; Protein: 11%; Carbs: 37%

AQUAFABA PER SERVING (3 TABLESPOONS): Calories: 8; Total Fat: 0g; Protein: 1g; Total carbs: 1g; Fiber: 0g; Net carbs: 1g

MACROS: Fat: 0%; Protein: 50%; Carbs: 50%

TIP: Whenever you use canned chickpeas, save the aquafaba by pouring it into an ice cube tray and freezing it (each cube is about 3 tablespoons of liquid). Whenever you need a vegan egg, just thaw 1 cube.

Tempeh "Bacon"

This wholesome approach to bacon is proof that spices and seasonings rule. Smoky, salty, and slightly sweet are the name of the game for a cured bacon–style flavor. Want a super-crispy vegan bacon with no frying? Pull out your air fryer and cook the tempeh at 330°F for 10 minutes, shaking the basket after 5 minutes. Raise the heat to 390°F and air-fry for 3 minutes more.

MAKES 8 SLICES • PREP TIME: 5 minutes • **COOK TIME:** 20 minutes

¼ cup Vegetable Broth (page 108) or store-bought vegetable broth

2 tablespoons pure maple syrup

1 teaspoon gluten-free soy sauce

½ teaspoon cayenne pepper

½ teaspoon smoked paprika

1 (8-ounce) package tempeh

1 Preheat the oven to 375°F. Line a baking sheet with parchment paper.

2 In a small bowl, whisk together the broth, maple syrup, soy sauce, cayenne, and paprika to create a marinade.

3 Cut the tempeh lengthwise into 8 slices. Place the slices on the prepared baking sheet. Drizzle half the marinade over the tempeh and spread it evenly with a basting brush.

4 Bake for 10 minutes, then flip the slices, brush the remaining marinade over the top, and bake for 8 minutes more.

5 Transfer the tempeh to a wire rack to cool. Serve immediately or store in the refrigerator for up to 5 days.

TIP: To make this bacon-style tempeh even more tender, place the tempeh in a resealable plastic bag. Combine the marinade ingredients in a measuring cup and pour the marinade into the bag. Seal the bag and turn it to coat the tempeh, then refrigerate overnight before baking.

PER SERVING (2 SLICES): Calories: 138; Total fat: 6g; Protein: 11g; Total carbs: 12g; Fiber: 0g; Net carbs: 12g

MACROS: Fat: 39%; Protein: 32%; Carbs: 29%

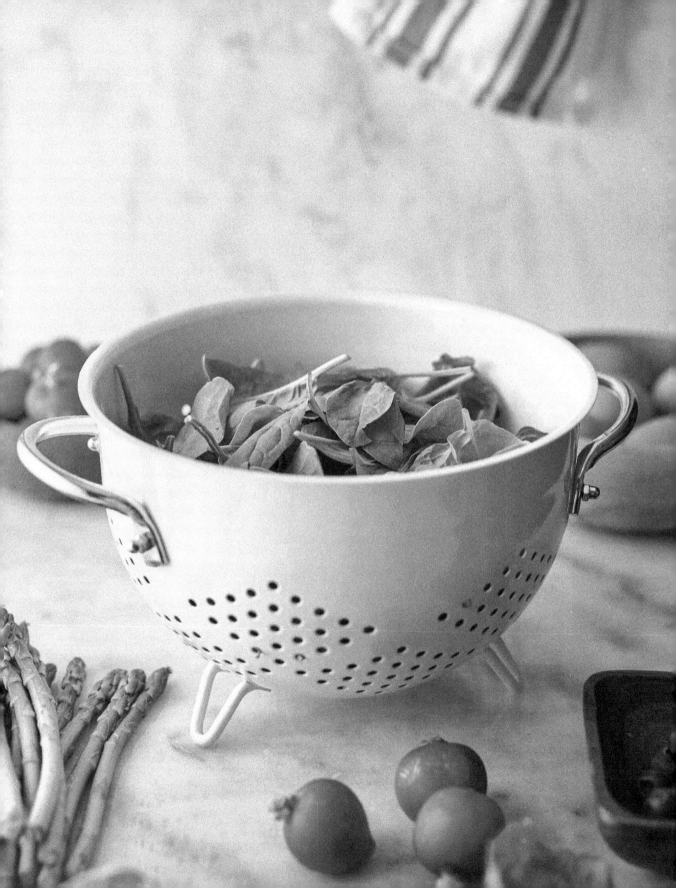

Measurement Conversions

VOLUME EQUIVALENTS (LIQUID)

US STANDARD	US STANDARD (OUNCES)	METRIC (APPROX.)
2 tablespoons	1 fl. oz.	30 mL
¼ cup	2 fl. oz.	60 mL
½ cup	4 fl. oz.	120 mL
1 cup	8 fl. oz.	240 mL
1½ cups	12 fl. oz.	355 mL
2 cups or 1 pint	16 fl. oz.	475 mL
4 cups or 1 quart	32 fl. oz.	1 L
1 gallon	128 fl. oz.	4 L

OVEN TEMPERATURES

FAHRENHEIT (F)	CELSIUS (C) (APPROX.)
250°	120°
300°	150°
325°	165°
350°	180°
375°	190°
400°	200°
425°	220°
450°	230°

VOLUME EQUIVALENTS (DRY)

US STANDARD	METRIC (APPROX.)
⅛ teaspoon	0.5 mL
¼ teaspoon	1 mL
½ teaspoon	2 mL
¾ teaspoon	4 mL
1 teaspoon	5 mL
1 tablespoon	15 mL
¼ cup	59 mL
⅓ cup	79 mL
½ cup	118 mL
⅔ cup	156 mL
¾ cup	177 mL
1 cup	235 mL
2 cups or 1 pint	475 mL
3 cups	700 mL
4 cups or 1 quart	1 L

WEIGHT EQUIVALENTS

US STANDARD	METRIC (APPROX.)
½ ounce	15 g
1 ounce	30 g
2 ounces	60 g
4 ounces	115 g
8 ounces	225 g
12 ounces	340 g
16 ounces or 1 pound	455 g

Index

A

Alcohol, 11
Almond Chocolate, Hot, 22
Aquafaba Eggs, 118
Asparagus and White Cheddar Soup, 52
Avocados
  Avocado Goddess Dressing, 115
  Cheese Chips & Guacamole, 85
  Chocolate Avocado Pudding, 98

B

Bacon
  "Bacon" Spinach Salad, 41
  "B"LT, 46
  Tempeh "Bacon," 119
Bagna Cauda Dip, 113
Balsamic Vinaigrette, 114
Basil
  Classic Pesto, 110
  Open-Faced Caprese Sandwich, 48
  Portabella Mushroom Margherita Pizza, 69
Berries
  Berry Cobbler, 104
  Blackberry "Cheesecake" Bites, 96
  Blackberry Cheesecake Smoothie, 25
  Raspberry Ice Cream, 99
Beverages, 12
  Bulletproof Coffee, 23
  Hot Almond Chocolate, 22
Bok Choy Ramen, Sesame, 58

Bread, Basic, 117
Breakfasts
  Brussel Browns, 28
  Cacao Crunch Cereal, 27
  Egg Muffins, 30
  French Toast Egg Loaf, 34
  Hazelnut "Sausage," 29
  Mushroom Feta Omelet, 31
  Shakshuka, 32–33
Broccoli Slaw, Ranch, 39
Broth, Vegetable, 108
Brussel Browns, 28
Buffalo "Mac-and-Cheese" Bake, 76
Bulletproof Coffee, 23

C

Cacao Crunch Cereal, 27
Caffeine, 12
Cakes, Carrot (Pan), 102–103
Carbohydrates, 4–6
Carrot (Pan)Cake, 102–103
Cauliflower
  Buffalo "Mac-and-Cheese" Bake, 76
  Cheesy Curried Cauliflower Chowder, 56–57
  Egg Cauliflower Tikka Masala, 81
  Garlic Fried Cauliflower Rice, 78
  Thai-Inspired Peanut Roasted
    Cauliflower, 80
Cayenne Pepper Vegetable Bake, 73
Cereal, Cacao Crunch, 27

Cheese
  Asparagus and White Cheddar Soup, 52
  Blackberry Cheesecake Smoothie, 25
  Buffalo "Mac-and-Cheese" Bake, 76
  Casserole Relleno, 77
  Cheese Chips & Guacamole, 85
  Cheesy Curried Cauliflower Chowder, 56–57
  Crustless Spanakopita, 70–71
  Fondue and Crudités, 87
  Mushroom Feta Omelet, 31
  Open-Faced Caprese Sandwich, 48
  Parmesan Radishes, 86
  Portabella Mushroom Margherita Pizza, 69
  Taco Tots and Dipping Sauce, 88–89
Chia Eggs, 118
Chiles, green
  Casserole Relleno, 77
  Green Chile Stew, 59
Chili Chocolate Fat Bombs, 92
Chimichurri, 112
Chipotle Chili, 60
Chocolate
  Chili Chocolate Fat Bombs, 92
  Chocolate Avocado Pudding, 98
  Chocolate Chip Bread, 117
  Chocolate Mint Smoothie, 26
  Cookie Fat Bombs, 91
  Hot Almond Chocolate, 22
  Morning Mocha Shake, 24
Coconut
  Coconut Leek Soup, 53
  Thai-Inspired Coconut Vegetable Soup, 54
Coffee, 12
  Bulletproof Coffee, 23
  Morning Mocha Shake, 24
Cookie Fat Bombs, 91
Cookies
  Peanut Butter Cookies, 100
  Pumpkin Spice Cookies, 101

D

Dairy-free. *See also* Vegan
  "Bacon" Spinach Salad, 41
  Berry Cobbler, 104

Brussel Browns, 28
Egg Foo Young, 79
Egg Muffins, 30
Egg White Salad, 44
Hazelnut "Sausage," 29
Peanut Butter Cookies, 100
Southwest Lettuce Cups, 45
Taco Slaw, 38
Desserts
  Berry Cobbler, 104
  Blackberry "Cheesecake" Bites, 96
  Carrot (Pan)Cake, 102–103
  Chocolate Avocado Pudding, 98
  Peanut Butter Cookies, 100
  Pumpkin Spice Cookies, 101
  Raspberry Ice Cream, 99
  Vanilla Pudding, 97
Dip, Bagna Cauda, 113
Dressings
  Avocado Goddess Dressing, 115
  Balsamic Vinaigrette, 114
  Ranch Dressing, 116

E

Egg-free
  Asparagus and White Cheddar Soup, 52
  Bagna Cauda Dip, 113
  Blackberry Cheesecake Smoothie, 25
  Buffalo "Mac-and-Cheese" Bake, 76
  Bulletproof Coffee, 23
  Cheese Chips & Guacamole, 85
  Cheesy Curried Cauliflower Chowder, 56–57
  Chocolate Mint Smoothie, 26
  Classic Pesto, 110
  Cream of Mushroom Soup, 55
  Fondue and Crudités, 87
  Hot Almond Chocolate, 22
  Morning Mocha Shake, 24
  Parmesan Radishes, 86
  Portabella Mushroom Margherita Pizza, 69
  Raspberry Ice Cream, 99
  Shirataki Florentine, 66
  Wild Mushroom Tofu Ragù, 68

Eggplants
   Eggplant Marinara, 67
   Ratatouille, 61
Eggs
   Egg Cauliflower Tikka Masala, 81
   Egg Foo Young, 79
   Egg Muffins, 30
   Egg White Salad, 44
   French Toast Egg Loaf, 34
   Mushroom Feta Omelet, 31
   Shakshuka, 32–33
   Spaghetti Squash Egg Bake, 74–75
Eggs, Vegan, Two Ways, 118
Exercise, 11

F

Fat bombs
   Chili Chocolate Fat Bombs, 92
   Cookie Fat Bombs, 91
Fats, 4–6
Fiber, 4
5-ingredient
   Asparagus and White Cheddar Soup, 52
   Bagna Cauda Dip, 113
   Balsamic Vinaigrette, 114
   Basic Bread, 117
   "B"LT, 46
   Brussel Browns, 28
   Bulletproof Coffee, 23
   Casserole Relleno, 77
   Cheese Chips & Guacamole, 85
   Chili Chocolate Fat Bombs, 92
   Chimichurri, 112
   Chocolate Avocado Pudding, 98
   Classic Pesto, 110
   Cookie Fat Bombs, 91
   Egg Muffins, 30
   Egg White Salad, 44
   French Toast Egg Loaf, 34
   Hot Almond Chocolate, 22
   Madeline's Marinade, 109
   Morning Mocha Shake, 24
   Parmesan Radishes, 86
   Peanut Butter Cookies, 100

Pico de Gallo, 111
Portabella Mushroom Margherita Pizza, 69
Ranch Broccoli Slaw, 39
Raspberry Ice Cream, 99
Vanilla Pudding, 97
Vegan Eggs, Two Ways, 118
Zucchini Chips, 84
Flax Eggs, 118
Fondue and Crudités, 87
French Toast Egg Loaf, 34

G

Garlic Fried Cauliflower Rice, 78
Glucose, 4
Gluten-free
   Asparagus and White Cheddar Soup, 52
   Avocado Goddess Dressing, 115
   "Bacon" Spinach Salad, 41
   Balsamic Vinaigrette, 114
   Basic Bread, 117
   Berry Cobbler, 104
   Blackberry "Cheesecake" Bites, 96
   Blackberry Cheesecake Smoothie, 25
   "B"LT, 46
   Brussel Browns, 28
   Bulletproof Coffee, 23
   Buon Gusto Salad, 40
   Cacao Crunch Cereal, 27
   Carrot (Pan)Cake, 102–103
   Casserole Relleno, 77
   Cayenne Pepper Vegetable Bake, 73
   Cheese Chips & Guacamole, 85
   Cheesy Curried Cauliflower Chowder, 56–57
   Chili Chocolate Fat Bombs, 92
   Chimichurri, 112
   Chipotle Chili, 60
   Chocolate Avocado Pudding, 98
   Chocolate Mint Smoothie, 26
   Classic Pesto, 110
   Coconut Leek Soup, 53
   Cookie Fat Bombs, 91
   Cream of Mushroom Soup, 55
   Crustless Spanakopita, 70–71
   Egg Cauliflower Tikka Masala, 81

Egg Foo Young, 79
Egg Muffins, 30
Eggplant Marinara, 67
Egg White Salad, 44
Fondue and Crudités, 87
French Toast Egg Loaf, 34
Garlic Fried Cauliflower Rice, 78
Gourmet "Cheese" Balls, 90
Green Bean and Mushroom
  Casserole, 72
Green Chile Stew, 59
Hazelnut "Sausage," 29
Hemp Cobb Salad, 43
Hot Almond Chocolate, 22
Madeline's Marinade, 109
Morning Mocha Shake, 24
Mushroom Feta Omelet, 31
Open-Faced Caprese Sandwich, 48
Parmesan Radishes, 86
Peanut Butter Cookies, 100
Pico de Gallo, 111
Portabella Mushroom Margherita
  Pizza, 69
Pumpkin Spice Cookies, 101
Ranch Broccoli Slaw, 39
Ranch Dressing, 116
Raspberry Ice Cream, 99
Ratatouille, 61
Ribollita, 62–63
Roasted Vegetable Wrap, 47
Shakshuka, 32–33
Shirataki Florentine, 66
Southwest Lettuce Cups, 45
Spaghetti Squash Egg Bake, 74–75
Taco Slaw, 38
Taco Tots and Dipping Sauce, 88–89
Tempeh "Bacon," 119
Thai-Inspired Coconut Vegetable
  Soup, 54
Thai-Inspired Peanut Roasted
  Cauliflower, 80
Vanilla Pudding, 97
Vegan Eggs, Two Ways, 118
Vegetable Broth, 108

Wild Mushroom Tofu Ragù, 68
Zucchini Chips, 84
Green Bean and Mushroom Casserole, 72
Guacamole, Cheese Chips &, 85

Hazelnut "Sausage," 29
Hemp Cobb Salad, 43

Ice Cream, Raspberry, 99
Intermittent fasting, 11

Keto flu, 10
Ketogenic diets
  foods to eat, 6–7
  frequently asked questions, 10–12
  how it works, 4–5
  meal plan, 12–19
  plant-based, 2
  tips, 3, 9
Ketosis, 4

Leek Soup, Coconut, 53
Lettuce
  "B"LT, 46
  Southwest Lettuce Cups, 45

Macronutrients, 4–5
Marinade, Madeline's, 109
Meal plan, 12–19
Micronutrients, 7
Mint Smoothie, Chocolate, 26
Mushrooms
  Cream of Mushroom Soup, 55
  Green Bean and Mushroom
    Casserole, 72
  Mushroom Feta Omelet, 31
  Portabella Mushroom Margherita
    Pizza, 69
  Wild Mushroom Tofu Ragù, 68

N

Noodles
  Sesame Bok Choy Ramen, 58
  Shirataki Florentine, 66
Nut-free
  Asparagus and White Cheddar Soup, 52
  Avocado Goddess Dressing, 115
  "Bacon" Spinach Salad, 41
  Bagna Cauda Dip, 113
  Balsamic Vinaigrette, 114
  "B"LT, 46
  Brussel Browns, 28
  Bulletproof Coffee, 23
  Buon Gusto Salad, 40
  Casserole Relleno, 77
  Cayenne Pepper Vegetable Bake, 73
  Cheese Chips & Guacamole, 85
  Cheesy Curried Cauliflower Chowder, 56–57
  Chimichurri, 112
  Chipotle Chili, 60
  Cream of Mushroom Soup, 55
  Egg Cauliflower Tikka Masala, 81
  Egg Foo Young, 79
  Egg White Salad, 44
  Fondue and Crudités, 87
  French Toast Egg Loaf, 34
  Garlic Fried Cauliflower Rice, 78
  Green Chile Stew, 59
  Hemp Cobb Salad, 43
  Madeline's Marinade, 109
  Mushroom Feta Omelet, 31
  Parmesan Radishes, 86
  Pico de Gallo, 111
  Portabella Mushroom Margherita Pizza, 69
  Ranch Dressing, 116
  Raspberry Ice Cream, 99
  Ratatouille, 61
  Roasted Vegetable Wrap, 47
  Sesame Bok Choy Ramen, 58
  Shakshuka, 32–33
  Shirataki Florentine, 66
  Spaghetti Squash Egg Bake, 74–75
  Taco Slaw, 38

  Tempeh "Bacon," 119
  Vanilla Pudding, 97
  Vegan Eggs, Two Ways, 118
  Vegetable Broth, 108
  Wild Mushroom Tofu Ragù, 68

O

One-pot
  Avocado Goddess Dressing, 115
  "Bacon" Spinach Salad, 41
  Bagna Cauda Dip, 113
  Balsamic Vinaigrette, 114
  Blackberry Cheesecake Smoothie, 25
  "B"LT, 46
  Bulletproof Coffee, 23
  Cacao Crunch Cereal, 27
  Cayenne Pepper Vegetable Bake, 73
  Chimichurri, 112
  Chipotle Chili, 60
  Chocolate Avocado Pudding, 98
  Chocolate Mint Smoothie, 26
  Classic Pesto, 110
  Coconut Leek Soup, 53
  Egg Cauliflower Tikka Masala, 81
  Green Bean and Mushroom Casserole, 72
  Hot Almond Chocolate, 22
  Madeline's Marinade, 109
  Morning Mocha Shake, 24
  Pico de Gallo, 111
  Ranch Broccoli Slaw, 39
  Ranch Dressing, 116
  Sesame Bok Choy Ramen, 58
  Shakshuka, 32–33
  Thai-Inspired Coconut Vegetable Soup, 54
  Vanilla Pudding, 97
  Vegan Eggs, Two Ways, 118
  Wild Mushroom Tofu Ragù, 68
  Zucchini Chips, 84

Pantry staples, 8–9
Peanut butter
  Peanut Butter Cookies, 100
  Thai-Inspired Peanut Roasted Cauliflower, 80

Pico de Gallo, 111
Pizza, Portabella Mushroom Margherita, 69
Proteins, 4–6
Puddings
  Chocolate Avocado Pudding, 98
  Vanilla Pudding, 97
Pumpkin Bread, 117
Pumpkin Spice Cookies, 101

Q

Quick
  Asparagus and White Cheddar Soup, 52
  Avocado Goddess Dressing, 115
  "Bacon" Spinach Salad, 41
  Bagna Cauda Dip, 113
  Balsamic Vinaigrette, 114
  Basic Bread, 117
  Blackberry Cheesecake Smoothie, 25
  "B"LT, 46
  Brussel Browns, 28
  Bulletproof Coffee, 23
  Buon Gusto Salad, 40
  Cacao Crunch Cereal, 27
  Carrot (Pan)Cake, 102–103
  Cheese Chips & Guacamole, 85
  Chili Chocolate Fat Bombs, 92
  Chimichurri, 112
  Chocolate Avocado Pudding, 98
  Chocolate Mint Smoothie, 26
  Classic Pesto, 110
  Cream of Mushroom Soup, 55
  Egg Muffins, 30
  Egg White Salad, 44
  Fondue and Crudités, 87
  French Toast Egg Loaf, 34
  Garlic Fried Cauliflower Rice, 78
  Green Chile Stew, 59
  Hazelnut "Sausage," 29
  Hemp Cobb Salad, 43
  Hot Almond Chocolate, 22
  Joe's Keto Salad, 42
  Madeline's Marinade, 109
  Morning Mocha Shake, 24
  Mushroom Feta Omelet, 31

Open-Faced Caprese Sandwich, 48
Peanut Butter Cookies, 100
Pico de Gallo, 111
Portabella Mushroom Margherita Pizza, 69
Pumpkin Spice Cookies, 101
Ranch Broccoli Slaw, 39
Ranch Dressing, 116
Roasted Vegetable Wrap, 47
Sesame Bok Choy Ramen, 58
Shirataki Florentine, 66
Southwest Lettuce Cups, 45
Taco Slaw, 38
Tempeh "Bacon," 119
Thai-Inspired Coconut Vegetable Soup, 54
Thai-Inspired Peanut Roasted Cauliflower, 80
Vegan Eggs, Two Ways, 118

R

Radishes, Parmesan, 86
Ratatouille, 61
Recipes, about, 13
Ribollita, 62–63

S

Salads
  "Bacon" Spinach Salad, 41
  Buon Gusto Salad, 40
  Egg White Salad, 44
  Hemp Cobb Salad, 43
  Joe's Keto Salad, 42
  Ranch Broccoli Slaw, 39
  Southwest Lettuce Cups, 45
  Taco Slaw, 38
Sandwiches and wraps
  "B"LT, 46
  Open-Faced Caprese Sandwich, 48
  Roasted Vegetable Wrap, 47
  Southwest Lettuce Cups, 45
Sauces
  Chimichurri, 112
  Classic Pesto, 110
  Pico de Gallo, 111
"Sausage," Hazelnut, 29
Sesame Bok Choy Ramen, 58

Shakshuka, 32–33
Smoothies and shakes
    Blackberry Cheesecake Smoothie, 25
    Chocolate Mint Smoothie, 26
    Morning Mocha Shake, 24
Snacks, 11–12
    Cheese Chips & Guacamole, 85
    Chili Chocolate Fat Bombs, 92
    Cookie Fat Bombs, 91
    Fondue and Crudités, 87
    Gourmet "Cheese" Balls, 90
    Parmesan Radishes, 86
    Taco Tots and Dipping Sauce, 88–89
    Zucchini Chips, 84
Soups, stews, and chilis
    Asparagus and White Cheddar Soup, 52
    Cheesy Curried Cauliflower Chowder, 56–57
    Chipotle Chili, 60
    Coconut Leek Soup, 53
    Cream of Mushroom Soup, 55
    Green Chile Stew, 59
    Ratatouille, 61
    Ribollita, 62–63
    Sesame Bok Choy Ramen, 58
    Thai-Inspired Coconut Vegetable Soup, 54
Soy-free
    Asparagus and White Cheddar Soup, 52
    Avocado Goddess Dressing, 115
    Balsamic Vinaigrette, 114
    Basic Bread, 117
    Berry Cobbler, 104
    Blackberry "Cheesecake" Bites, 96
    Blackberry Cheesecake Smoothie, 25
    Brussel Browns, 28
    Buffalo "Mac-and-Cheese" Bake, 76
    Bulletproof Coffee, 23
    Cacao Crunch Cereal, 27
    Carrot (Pan)Cake, 102–103
    Casserole Relleno, 77
    Cayenne Pepper Vegetable Bake, 73
    Cheese Chips & Guacamole, 85
    Cheesy Curried Cauliflower Chowder, 56–57
    Chili Chocolate Fat Bombs, 92

Chimichurri, 112
Chipotle Chili, 60
Chocolate Avocado Pudding, 98
Chocolate Mint Smoothie, 26
Classic Pesto, 110
Cookie Fat Bombs, 91
Cream of Mushroom Soup, 55
Crustless Spanakopita, 70–71
Egg Cauliflower Tikka Masala, 81
Egg Foo Young, 79
Egg Muffins, 30
Eggplant Marinara, 67
Egg White Salad, 44
Fondue and Crudités, 87
French Toast Egg Loaf, 34
Green Bean and Mushroom Casserole, 72
Green Chile Stew, 59
Hazelnut "Sausage," 29
Hot Almond Chocolate, 22
Joe's Keto Salad, 42
Madeline's Marinade, 109
Morning Mocha Shake, 24
Mushroom Feta Omelet, 31
Open-Faced Caprese Sandwich, 48
Parmesan Radishes, 86
Peanut Butter Cookies, 100
Pico de Gallo, 111
Portabella Mushroom Margherita Pizza, 69
Pumpkin Spice Cookies, 101
Ranch Broccoli Slaw, 39
Ranch Dressing, 116
Raspberry Ice Cream, 99
Ratatouille, 61
Ribollita, 62–63
Roasted Vegetable Wrap, 47
Shakshuka, 32–33
Shirataki Florentine, 66
Southwest Lettuce Cups, 45
Spaghetti Squash Egg Bake, 74–75
Taco Tots and Dipping Sauce, 88–89
Thai-Inspired Coconut Vegetable Soup, 54
Thai-Inspired Peanut Roasted Cauliflower, 80
Vanilla Pudding, 97

Vegan Eggs, Two Ways, 118
Vegetable Broth, 108
Zucchini Chips, 84
Spaghetti Squash Egg Bake, 74–75
Spinach
    "Bacon" Spinach Salad, 41
    Crustless Spanakopita, 70–71
    Shirataki Florentine, 66
Supplements, 11

T

Taco Slaw, 38
Taco Tots and Dipping Sauce, 88–89
Tea, 12
Tempeh "Bacon," 119
Tofu Ragù, Wild Mushroom, 68
Tomatoes
    "B"LT, 46
    Open-Faced Caprese Sandwich, 48
    Pico de Gallo, 111
    Portabella Mushroom Margherita Pizza, 69
    Shakshuka, 32–33
Tools, 10

V

Vanilla Pudding, 97
Vegan
    Avocado Goddess Dressing, 115
    Balsamic Vinaigrette, 114
    Blackberry "Cheesecake" Bites, 96
    Cacao Crunch Cereal, 27
    Cayenne Pepper Vegetable Bake, 73
    Chili Chocolate Fat Bombs, 92

Chimichurri, 112
Chipotle Chili, 60
Chocolate Avocado Pudding, 98
Coconut Leek Soup, 53
Cookie Fat Bombs, 91
Garlic Fried Cauliflower Rice, 78
Gourmet "Cheese" Balls, 90
Green Bean and Mushroom
    Casserole, 72
Green Chile Stew, 59
Madeline's Marinade, 109
Pico de Gallo, 111
Ratatouille, 61
Roasted Vegetable Wrap, 47
Sesame Bok Choy Ramen, 58
Tempeh "Bacon," 119
Thai-Inspired Coconut Vegetable Soup, 54
Thai-Inspired Peanut Roasted Cauliflower, 80
Vegan Eggs, Two Ways, 118
Vegetable Broth, 108
Zucchini Chips, 84
Vegetables. *See also specific*
    Cayenne Pepper Vegetable Bake, 73
    Fondue and Crudités, 87
    Roasted Vegetable Wrap, 47
    Taco Tots and Dipping Sauce, 88–89
    Thai-Inspired Coconut Vegetable Soup, 54
    Vegetable Broth, 108

Z

Zucchini
    Ratatouille, 61
    Zucchini Chips, 84

Acknowledgments

My deepest gratitude for contributions large and small go to:

Mark, my best friend, for embracing the joy and silliness of our everyday life.

Celeste, my mother, for showing me the glory of celebration and the power of restraint.

My family, for understanding that my love for our heritage has no bounds.

My friends, for knowing the perfect emojis to text, no matter the occasion.

The Dinkdom, for reading, liking, and commenting.

I love you all.

About the Author

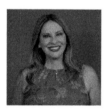

Alicia Shevetone is an energetic culinary personality, cookbook author, and creator of Dink Cuisine, a food and entertainment organization that promotes cooking experiences across print, digital, social, and live media. Shevetone encourages people to come together in the kitchen, look at cooking as a creative and fun activity to share with those they're closest to, and enjoy the process. She is passionate about living a balanced life with her husband (Mark) and English Bulldog (Belma), creating unique and delicious low-carb recipes, and reinventing humble foods in uncommonly savory ways.

The following authors also contributed recipes to this book: Jen Fish (*Keto in 30 Minutes*), Brian Stanton and Michelle Anderson (*Keto Intermittent Fasting*), Molly Devine, RD (*The Essential Ketogenic Mediterranean Diet Cookbook*), Lisa Danielson (*Keto for Vegetarians*), Nicole Derseweh and Whitney Lauritsen (*The Vegan Ketogenic Diet Cookbook*), Jessica Dukes (*The Dairy-Free Ketogenic Diet Cookbook*), and JL Fields (*The Complete Plant-Based Diet*).

CPSIA information can be obtained
at www.ICGtesting.com
Printed in the USA
JSHW051912130122
21967JS00002B/15

9 781638 073086